CW00542155

SELF-ASSESSMENT P1
VETERINARY 1

SMALL ANIMAL PRACTICE

Edited by
R. D. Long, BVetMed, Cert V Ophthal, MRCVS
Stone Lion Veterinary Hospital
London, England

Wolfe Publishing Ltd

Copyright © Wolfe Publishing Ltd.
Published by Wolfe Publishing Ltd, 1992.
Printed by BPCC Hazell Books, Aylesbury, England
ISBN 0 7234 1745 8

A CIP catalogue record for this book is available from the
British Library.

For full details of all Wolfe titles please write to
Wolfe Publishing Ltd, Brook House, 2–16 Torrington Place,
London WC1E 7LT, England.

PREFACE

'Experience is as to intensity not duration'.
Thomas Hardy

We all have to work at keeping abreast of the knowledge available, and experience does not necessarily come with age alone. The intensity with which we apply ourselves produces much more experience than does the passing of time.

This series of questions and answers, is designed for students and practitioners, and is meant to assist in the assimilation of knowledge. The contributors are recognised specialists in their fields and the questions they have produced cover the broad spectrum of Small Animal Practice. Their answers are especially educational and thought provoking. It is hoped that the random nature of the sequence of questions will maintain interest, and yet make it possible to work through the book in small bites between meals, with the answers being chewed over and digested at will.

Raymond D. Long

ACKNOWLEDGEMENTS

P. Holt acknowledges, with thanks, M. Parsons and J. Conibear for photographic assistance, and the Editor of *In Practice* for permission to reproduce figures.

LIST OF CONTRIBUTORS

W.E. Allen, MVB, PhD, FRCVS, Department of Veterinary Surgery and Obstetrics, Royal Veterinary College, Hatfield, Hertfordshire, England

K.C. Barnett, MA, PhD, BSc, FRCVS, DV Ophthal, Comparative Ophthalmology Unit, Animal Health Trust, Newmarket, Suffolk, England

S.E. Brownlie, BVM&S, PhD, MRCVS, Cert SAC, Department of Medicine, Royal Veterinary College, Hatfield, Hertfordshire, England

K.W. Clarke, MA, VetMB, DVetMed, MRCVS, Department of Surgery, Royal Veterinary College, Hatfield, Hertfordshire, England

J.E. Cooper, BVSc, FRCVS, FIBiol, MRC Path, DTVM, Royal College of Surgeons of England, London, England

R. Dennis, MA, VetMB, DVR, MRCVS, Department of Clinical Veterinary Medicine, University of Cambridge, Cambridge, England

C.J. Gaskell, BVSc, PhD, DVR, MRCVS, University of Liverpool Small Animal Hospital, Liverpool, England

M.E. Herrtage, MA, BVSc, DVR, DVD, MRCVS, Department of Clinical Veterinary Medicine, University of Cambridge, Cambridge, England

P.E. Holt, BVM&S, PhD, FIBiol, MIBiol, MRCVS, Department of Veterinary Surgery, University of Bristol, Bristol, England

J.E.F. Houlton, MA, VetMB, DSAO, DVR, MRCVS, Surgery Division, Department of Clinical Veterinary Medicine, University of Cambridge Veterinary School, Cambridge, England

M. G. Kerr, BVM&S, BSc, PhD, MRCVS, Vetlab Services, Horsham, Sussex, England

P. Kertesz, BDS, LDS, RCS(Eng), 29a Brook Street, London, England

J. G. Lane, BVetMed, FRCVS, Department of Veterinary Surgery, University of Bristol School of Veterinary Science, Bristol, England.

D.H. Scarff, BVetMed, MRCVS, Cert.SAD, Department of Veterinary Surgery and Obstetrics, Royal Veterinary College, London, England

R.A.S. White, BVetMed, PhD, DVR, FRCVS, Department of Clinical Veterinary Medicine, University of Cambridge, Cambridge, England

1 The cat in *Figure 1* has had this apparently non-pruritic lesion for 3 weeks.
(a) What are the differential diagnoses?
(b) How could you confirm the diagnosis?
(c) Are there any public health implications?

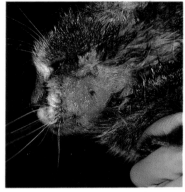

Figure 1

2 A 7-year-old male Dobermann Pinscher has had several days' treatment for cardiac failure but his condition has suddenly worsened.
(a) How would you report the ECG (*Figure 2*)?
(b) What might be the cause of the deterioration?

Figure 2

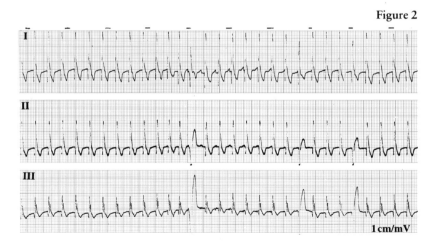

1 cm/mV

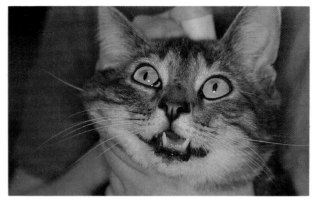

Figure 3

3   This cat (*Figure 3*) returned from a night out unable to eat normally.
(a) What injury has been sustained?
(b) What are the anatomical principles involved in its correction?

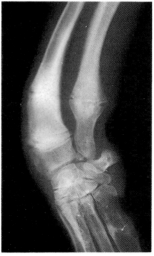

4   The puppy in *Figure 4* fractured its foreleg 3 weeks previously.
(a) What is the diagnosis?
(b) What clinical signs are likely to develop?
(c) How would you treat this dog?

Figure 4

5   List the major criteria that influence your choice of exposure factors when taking X-rays.

6 A middle-aged Samoyed is presented with a persistent ocular discharge (*Figure 5*) of several weeks' duration.
(a) What is your diagnosis?
(b) What features lead you to this diagnosis?
(c) How would you confirm this diagnosis?

Figure 5

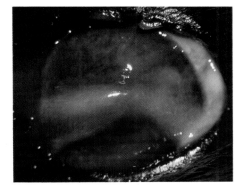

7 Comment on the procedure shown in *Figure 6*.

Figure 6

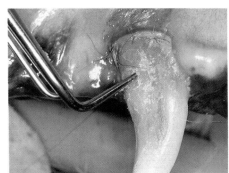

8 A 9-year-old cat is presented with lameness in the left forelimb which has been obvious for some months and is getting worse. The elbow joint is swollen and restricted in movement, but not hot. The cat continues to eat well, has not lost weight, but is 'grumpy'. A radiograph is made (*Figure 7*). What is your diagnosis?

Figure 7

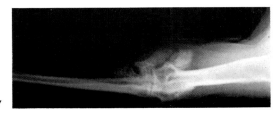

9 A 12-year-old neutered cross-bred dog was presented with a complaint of severe vomiting for the previous 36 hours. An accurate history was difficult to obtain as the elderly owner was somewhat confused, but it appeared that no abnormalities had been noted prior to the onset of the vomiting, and no diarrhoea had been seen. On examination the dog appeared dull and depressed, and he had several attacks of retching while in the consulting room. A small amount of bilious fluid was produced. He was underweight, with ribs and spinous processes readily palpable, and appeared moderately dehydrated. The teeth were badly encrusted with tartar. The abdomen was tense and difficult to palpate, but no abnormalities were palpable so far as could be ascertained. Rectal temperature was 38.4°C.
(a) What are the main differential diagnoses at this stage?
(b) What tests should be carried out to investigate these possibilities further?
A plain lateral X-ray film of the abdomen revealed no abnormalities, and it was decided not to attempt a barium series at this stage due to the severity of the vomiting. Biochemistry and haematology results are given in *Table 1*.

Table 1

Total protein	81g/l	(55–75)
Albumin	37g/l	(25–35)
Globulin	44g/l	(30–40)
Na$^+$	154mmol/l	(140–155)
K$^+$	3.2mmol/l	(3.5–5.5)
Urea	96.4 mmol	(2–8)
Creatinine	897μmol/l	(<120)
ALT	72iu/l	(<100)
ALP	43iu/l	(<300)
Amylase	5126iu/l	(<3000)
Lipase	245iu/l	(300)
PCV	0.31	(0.35–0.60)
MCV	66fl	(65–80)
MCHC	32.1g/100 ml	(30–40)
Total white cell count	21.6×10^9/l	(5–14)
Band neutrophils	0.6×10^9/l	(<1)
Adult neutrophils	17.0×10^9/l	(4–10)
Eosinophils	0.3×10^9/l	(<1)
Lymphocytes	2.6×10^9/^{1}	(1–5)
Monocytes	1.1×10^9/l	(<0.5)

RBC picture was non-regenerative and normochromic. No abnormal WBCs were seen.
(c) What is your diagnosis, and is the condition acute or chronic?
(d) How do the white cell abnormalities and the amylase result relate to the diagnosis?
(e) What is the prognosis?

10 *Figure 8* shows circuit diagrams of four non-rebreathing anaesthetic circuits (and one adaption) commonly used in small animal practices.
(a) Name these circuits.
(b) With each, what flow rates of gas (oxygen plus nitrous oxide, if in use) are used to prevent rebreathing?
(c) Which circuit would you use to anaesthetise:
  (i) A 3 kg cat?
  (ii) A 20 kg dog?

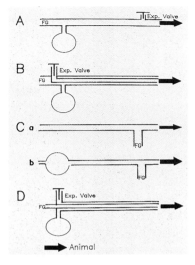

Figure 8

11 (a) What urological procedure has been performed on this male dog (*Figure 9*)?
(b) Give two indications for this procedure and two potential post-operative complications.

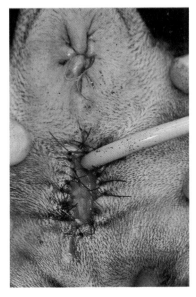

Figure 9

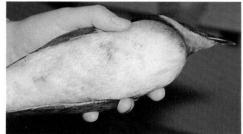

Figure 10

12 *Figure 10* shows a guillemot (Uria aalge) rescued from an oil slick.
(a) How severely is it affected?
(b) What treatment would you give?

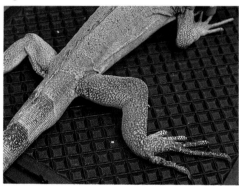

Figure 11

13 (a) What do you notice about the iguana (Iguana iguana) in *Figure 11*, which was presented for examination on account of lameness?
(b) List possible diagnoses.

14 Your practice has recently acquired a real-time B-mode ultrasound scanner suitable for pregnancy diagnosis in the bitch. What service will you offer to your dog-breeding clients?

15 You are presented with a 14-week-old bitch which has a creamy vulval discharge (*Figure 12*) causing matting of the perivulval hair.
(a) What is your diagnosis?
(b) How would you treat the condition?

Figure 12

16 A rabbit was treated for 3 days with an oral antibiotic. At post-mortem examination the stomach revealed the lesions seen in *Figure 13*.
(a) What is your diagnosis?
(b) What lesson can be learned from this case?

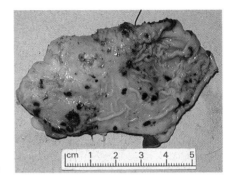

Figure 13

17 What are your comments on the budgerigar (Melopsittacus undulatus), illustrated in *Figure 14*, and presented for a health check?

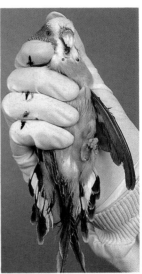

18 Is benign hormonal enlargement of the canine prostate gland always due to a relative excess of androgens?

Figure 14

19 Halothane, methoxyflurane and isoflurane are volatile anaesthetic agents which are used in dogs and cats. Which of these three drugs:
(a) Gives the fastest induction?
(b) Gives the fastest recovery?
(c) Is the best analgesic?
(d) Causes most respiratory depression?
(e) Causes least hypotension?
(f) Causes most myocardial depression?

20 A 9-year-old cross-bred bitch was presented with a complaint of polydipsia and polyuria, which had been noticed for at least 2 months and was gradually increasing in severity. The bitch was otherwise bright with a good appetite, but the owners complained that her coat was dull and lifeless, and thin in patches. There was no pruritus. Although she had not been spayed, she had not been seen in season for at least a year. On examination the skin was noticed to be rather thin and wrinkled, the dry hair was easily pulled out by the roots, and thinning of the coat was evident – especially in the groin and axilla. Body condition was fair to good, but a degree of abdominal enlargement was present, with palpable hepatomegaly. No enlarged uterus was palpable and there was no vulval discharge.

(a) What is the most probable provisional diagnosis?

Routine biochemistry and haematology based on the differential diagnosis of causes of polydipsia were carried out, and the results are given in *Table 2*.

Table 2

Total protein	65g/l	(55–75)
Albumin	28g/l	(25–35)
Globulin	37g/l	(30–40
Calcium	2.16mmol/l	(2.0–3.0)
Urea	2.1mmol/l	(2–8)
Creatinine	84μmol/l	(<120)
Glucose	5.2mmol/l	(4–6)
Cholesterol	9.6mmol/l	(2.5–7.5)
ALT	102iu/l	(<100)
ALP	1136iu/l	(<300)
PCV	0.56	(0.35–0.60)
MCV	76fl	(65–80)
MCHC	32.1g/100 ml	(30–40)
Total white cell count	10.2×10^9/l	(5–14)
Adult neutrophils	8.0×10^9/l	(4–10)
Eosinophils	0.1×10^9/l	(<1)
Lymphocytes	1.2×10^9/l	(1–5)
Monocytes	0.9×10^9/l	(<0.5)

RBC picture was moderately regenerative and no abnormal WBCs were seen.

(b) List the features that might be seen on the above 'profile' which would substantiate the provisional diagnosis.

(c) Which of the features are present in this case?

(d) Is this sufficient to continue with the current line of investigation?

(e) What further investigation(s) is/are necessary to establish the diagnosis with certainty?

(f) Why is such investigation essential, rather than instituting treatment on a 'see what happens' basis?

21 An 18-month-old Lurcher bitch is presented with a chronic cough. The owner acquired the bitch 4 months ago from 'a friend who keeps a few'; the dog has coughed ever since he bought it, but is otherwise well. It is keen to exercise but 'gets a bit out of breath and starts coughing' when run hard.
(a) What is your tentative diagnosis?
(b) How might this be confirmed and treated?

22 (a) What is the name of the structure indicated in *Figure 15*?
(b) What is its significance?

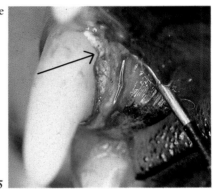

Figure 15

23 A 1-year-old golden retriever (*Figure 16*) has developed a total opacity in one eye, and on examination a partial opacity is found to be present in the other eye.
(a) What is your diagnosis?
(b) What other breed shows this type of inherited condition?
(c) What is your advice to the owner?

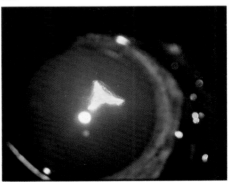

Figure 16

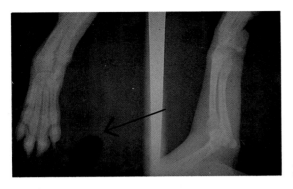

Figure 17

24 (a) What test is being performed here (*Figure 17*).
(b) Which radiographic fault does it detect?
(c) How may that fault be avoided?

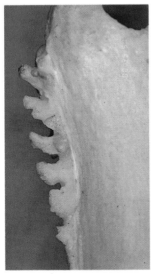

25 (a) Describe the periosteal reaction apparent in *Figure 18*.
(b) In what condition does this typically occur?
(c) What are the usual clinical features of this condition?

Figure 19

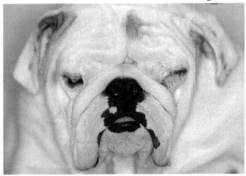

Figure 18

26 How many different forms of airway obstruction might afflict a 12-month-old English bulldog (*Figure 19*), and can you list them?

Figure 20

27 An 8-year-old cross-bred dog has ascites and slight subcutaneous oedema.
(a) What is your interpretation of the short axis view across the ventricles seen in the first ultrasound image (*Figure 20*).
(b) What is your interpretation of the long axis view of the left ventricular outflow tract (*Figure 21*)?

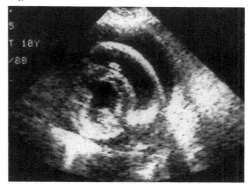

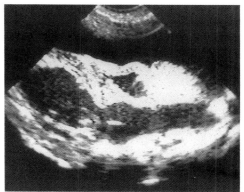

Figure 21

28 These hairs (*Figure 22*) have been taken from a young stray female domestic long-hair cat with a generalised scaling and crusting condition.
(a) What is the likely aetiology?
(b) How would you manage this condition?
(c) What complications could arise with systemic treatment in this cat?
(d) How might you reduce the zoonotic potential in this case?

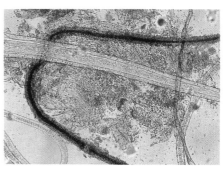

Figure 22

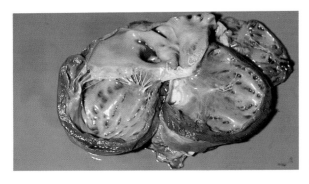

Figure 23

29 This post-mortem specimen (*Figure 23*) taken from a 2-year-old Great Dane which died suddenly, is laid out to show the left side of the heart. What are your observations?

30 (a) What is the likely diagnosis in *Figure 24* (a dog's elbow)?
(b) What are the pathological changes?
(c) What are the complications of surgery? (*Figure 25*)

Figure 24

Figure 25

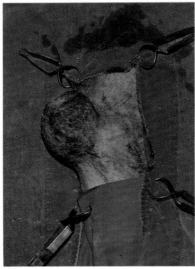

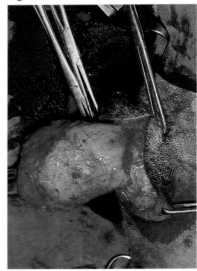

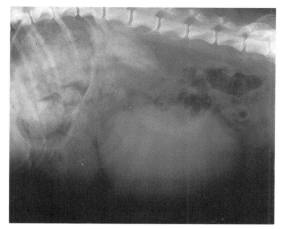

Figure 26

31 A 12-year-old Labrador is described as having 'put on weight' at a routine vaccination. The abdomen is distended and palpation reveals a firm ventral abdominal mass. A lateral abdominal radiograph is taken (*Figure 26*). What is your diagnosis?

32 (a) What other names have been used to describe feline cervical resorption (*Figure 27*)?
(b) Does the condition have a clinical significance?
(c) What is the most predictable treatment?

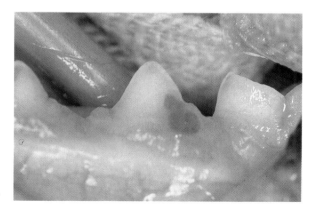

Figure 27

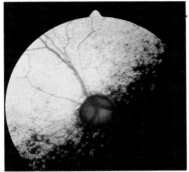

Figure 28

33 *Figure 28* shows the retina of a 2-year-old Toy poodle.
(a) Is the retina normal?
(b) What is/are the distinguishing ophthalmoscopic features?

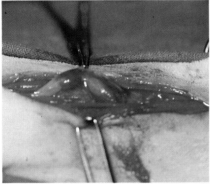

Figure 29

34 Thyroidectomy is generally considered to be the most practicable method to treat feline hyperthyroidism, and when both glands are hypertrophied (adenomatous) bilateral thyroidectomy is advocated. *Figure 29* depicts the surgery in progress.
(a) What are the common complications of this surgery?
(b) How can they be avoided?

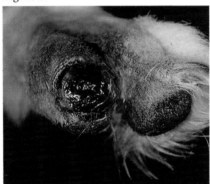

Figure 30

35 An 8-year-old golden retriever is presented with a history of pain involving the digit shown in *Figure 30*.
(a) What is the differential diagnosis?
(b) How might you try to confirm your diagnosis?
(c) How would you manage either condition?
(d) What is the prognosis for the two differentials?

36 Which of the following is/are associated with dietary taurine deficiency in the cat?
(a) Central retinal degeneration.
(b) Hepatic lipidosis.
(c) Cardiomyopathy.
(d) Seborrhoea.
(e) Aortic thromboembolism.

37 A bitch is presented with chronic perivulval irritation which stimulates constant licking and discomfort (*Figure 31*).
(a) What is the probable cause?
(b) How may it be treated?

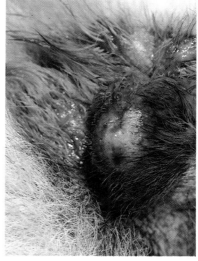

Figure 31

38 The swab being taken from a purulent lesion in an anaesthetised rabbit (Oryctolagus cuniculus) in *Figure 32* yielded *Pasteurella multocida*.
(a) What is your diagnosis?
(b) How would you treat the animal?

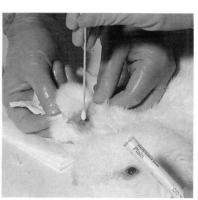

Figure 32

39 A cat with a fractured femur was anaesthetised. Induction was with thiopentone (*thiopental*), intubation with a 5mm uncuffed endotracheal tube, and maintenance was with methoxyflurane. Half-an-hour after the end of anaesthesia the cat had not recovered consciousness.
(a) Why may this have happened?
(b) What would you do?

40 An 11-year-old spayed female Boxer was presented with a complaint of intermittent vomiting with apparent abdominal pain. Further questioning of the owner revealed that there was also a recent history of weight loss and mild polydipsia. On clinical examination the bitch was fairly bright and in fair bodily condition. Numerous nodular skin tumours were evident scattered around the body, with several on the face. Rectal temperature was 38.4°C, heart and respiratory rates, and chest auscultation, were all normal. Abdominal palpation was extremely difficult, as the bitch tensed her muscles very markedly whenever the area was touched. The impression given was that of pain in the abdomen. As a consequence of certain suspicious-looking cells seen on haematological examination a buffy coat smear was prepared. *Figure 33* shows a representative field.
(a) What is the purpose of a buffy coat smear?
(b) What is the main (diagnostic) abnormality visible in *Figure 33*?
(c) What is your diagnosis?
(d) What is the prognosis?

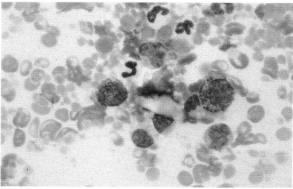

Figure 33

41 The tarantula (Eurypelma vagans) in *Figure 34* appeared lethargic and had bare areas on its abdomen. Comment on these features and what you see in the picture.

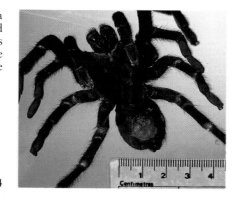

Figure 34

42 (a) What clinical sign is the juvenile golden retriever in *Figure 35* exhibiting?
(b) List five conditions which may result in this sign.
(c) Suggest two radiographic techniques which could be used to investigate this case further.

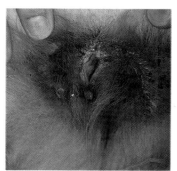

Figure 35

43 A 4-year-old oestrous bitch is presented with a large oedematous mass protruding from her vulva (*Figure 36*). The mass has grown rapidly in size over the preceding 5 days.
(a) What is the likely diagnosis?
(b) How might you manage this case?

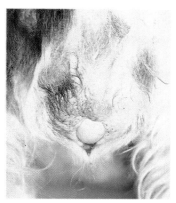

Figure 36

44 Shortly after moving house, a family consulted their new veterinary surgeon with a complaint that their 18-month-old Labrador cross dog had begun behaving strangely, crying persistently for no reason, wandering restlessly around the house and sitting staring at blank walls. Records forwarded by the previous veterinary surgeon indicated that the dog had been investigated about 9 months previously for poor weight gain and chronic unthriftiness. Exocrine pancreatic insufficiency (EPI) had been diagnosed and treated with pancreatic supplementation. The biochemistry results on which this was based are given in *Table 3*.

Table 3

Total protein	55g/l	(55–75)
Albumin	21g/l	(25–35)
Globulin	34g/l	(30–40)
Urea	2.3mmol	(2–8)
Creatinine	47μmol/l	(<120)
ALT	114iu/l	(<100)
ALP	346iu/l	(<300)
Bile acids	814μmol/l	(<10)
IRT (TLI)	4.9ng/ml	(>5.0)

(a) What is your comment on the diagnosis of EPI? ('This is usually associated with carcinoma of the liver' was the laboratory's annotation of the very high bile acid result. As this seemed highly unlikely in a 9-month-old pup, the figure was ignored by the practice.)
(b) Comment on the likely significance of such a result in a dog of this age. What is the probable diagnosis?
(c) What tests should be carried out to confirm this?

The routine biochemistry tests were repeated, with broadly similar results to the earlier occasion. Results of additional tests are given in *Table 4*.

Table 4

Ammonia	310μmol/l	(<60)
Fasting bile acids	25μmol/l	(<10)
Post-feeding bile acids	286μmol/l	(<15)

(d) Does the above confirm your diagnosis?
(e) What is the reason for the extremely large increase in bile acids after feeding that is experienced in this condition?
(f) What is the next stage in investigation/treatment?
(g) What is the prognosis?

45 (a) What is the likely cause of the lesions in this budgerigar (*Figure 37*)?
(b) How would you confirm your diagnosis?

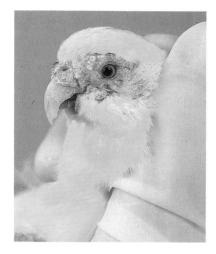

Figure 37

46 Which of the following is/are useful in treating the metabolic consequences of bladder rupture?
(a) Intravenous fluid therapy.
(b) Intravenous sodium bicarbonate.
(c) In dwelling catheterisation of the bladder.
(d) Abdominal drainage and peritoneal dialysis.

47 *Figure 38* illustrates the vulva of a female ferret.
(a) What is a female ferret called?
(b) What is the significance of a vulval swelling in this species?

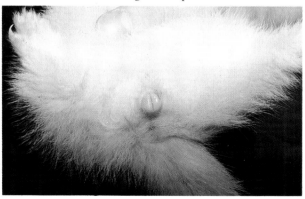

Figure 38

48 (a) What parameters should be observed constantly throughout anaesthesia?
(b) In the absence of sophisticated equipment how may such parameters be monitored?
(c) For which parameters do you consider the use of monitoring apparatus to be a priority?

49 This puppy (*Figure 39*) has a congenital stifle deformity and is unable to extend either joint fully.
(a) What is the likely condition?
(b) List the possible bony deformities.
(c) In which breeds does the condition usually occur?

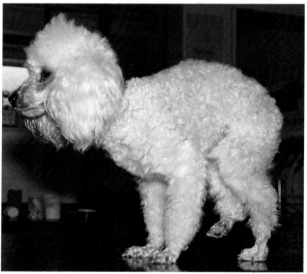

Figure 39

50 A dog was presented with abdominal distension (*Figure 40*) 4 days after being hit by a car. Paracentesis (*Figure 41*) recovered copious amounts of dark green/brown fluid (*Figure 42*).
(a) What diagnostic steps should be carried out on the fluid?
(b) What is the likely source of the fluid?
(c) What surgical procedures(s) should be performed to correct the accumulation of the fluid?
(d) What are the possible complications of the surgical procedure(s) that you describe?

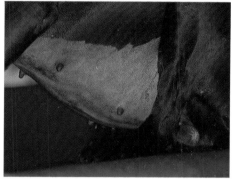

Figure 40

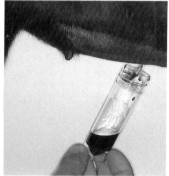

Figure 41

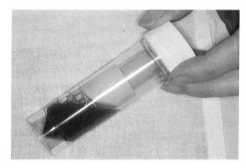

Figure 42

51 (a) What is the condition illustrated in *Figure 43* called?
(b) What is the likely pathology?
(c) How does this injury differ from a 'dropped toe'?

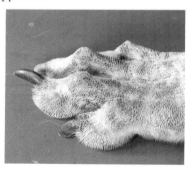

Figure 43

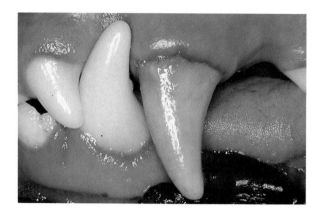

Figure 44

52 (a) What has caused the discolouration of the upper canine seen in *Figure 44*?
(b) What other colours may be demonstrated?
(c) What is the treatment of choice?

53 A 9-year-old German shepherd dog has become increasingly lethargic over a 3-week period, a sudden onset of blindness ensuing. When examined, the dog will walk but is difficult to arouse. The heart rate is very slow.
(a) How would you interpret the ECG pictured in *Figure 45*?
(b) What is the significance of this finding in relation to the clinical signs?

Figure 45

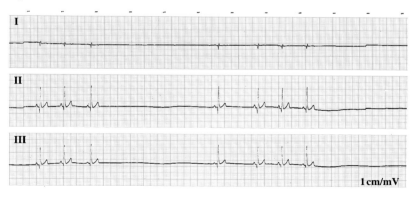

54 (a) Describe the radiographic changes apparent in *Figure 46* and name the condition.
(b) What are the usual haematological and biochemical findings in this condition?
(c) Which breed of dog is most commonly affected?

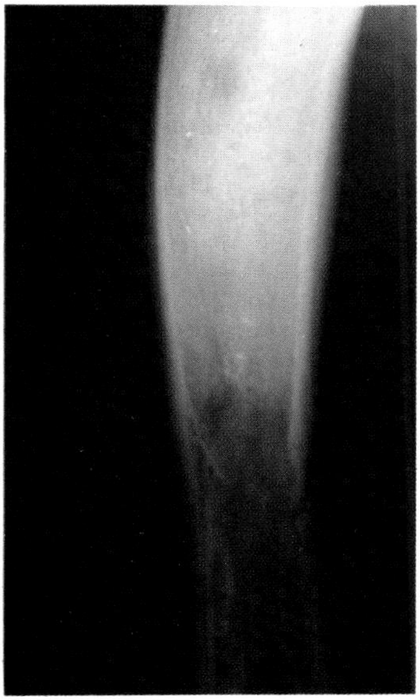

55 *Figure 47* illustrates positive contrast retrograde urethrocystogram in a juvenile West Highland white terrier dog.
(a) What has happened and what is the cause?
(b) What pre-existing condition may have predisposed these events?

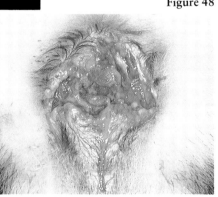

Figure 46

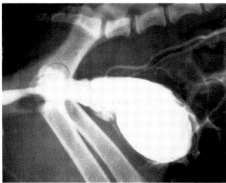

Figure 48

Figure 47

56 This German shepherd dog (*Figure 48*) has exhibited pain on defecation for several months, together with an increased interest in the perianal area.
(a) What is your diagnosis?
(b) How is this condition best treated?
(c) What is the prognosis?

27

Figure 49

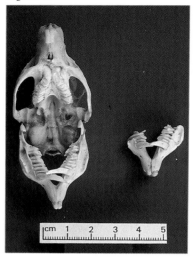

57 (a) Describe the changes in these guinea pig skulls (*Figure 49*).
(b) Are the lesions due to:
    (i) An infectious agent?
    (ii) A nutritional deficiency?
    (iii) A genetic factor?
    (iv) None of the above?

58 A dog owner asks you to terminate the unwanted pregnancy resulting from an inadvertent mating involving his bitch. What options are available?

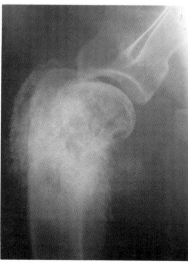

59 A 6-year-old Great Dane bitch is presented with a worsening right foreleg lameness of 2 weeks duration. There is marked muscle wastage and pain on palpation of the shoulder. A lateral radiograph of the affected joint is taken (*Figure 50*). A proximal portion of the humerus is surrounded by a florid periosteal reaction up to 2 cm deep, extending a considerable distance distally along the humeral shaft. Small irregular areas of osteolysis are also visible, especially in the metaphysis and greater tubercle. The cortex is thinned in places and subtle osteolysis extends distally. The articular surface of the humerus and the scapula is unaffected. What is your diagnosis?

Figure 50

60 (a) What is your diagnosis of the dog depicted in *Figure 51*?
(b) What is the likely cause?
(c) What treatment is indicated?

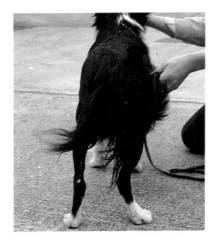

Figure 51

61 A 9-year-old German shepherd dog is presented for ECG following two episodes of collapse with pale mucous membranes. The dog was very depressed for 24 hours after each episode but soon returned to normal.
(a) How would you interpret the ECG (*Figure 52*)?
(b) What would you do next?

Figure 52

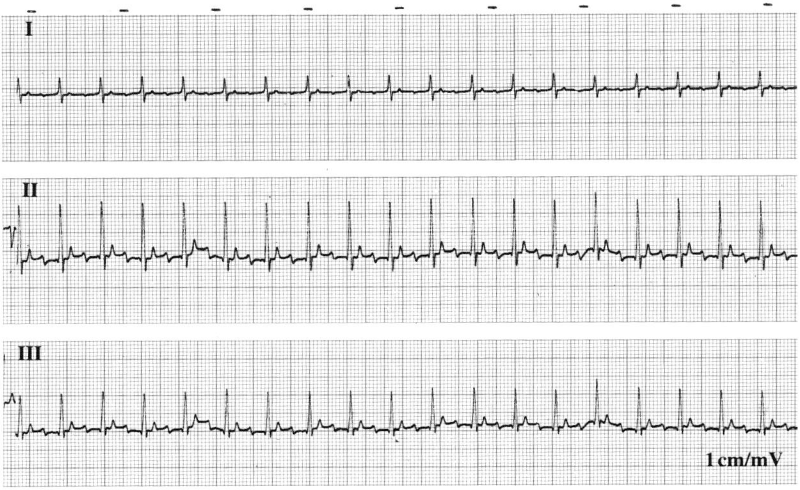

I

II

III

1 cm/mV

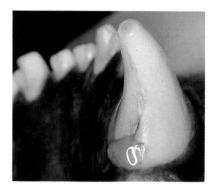

Figure 53

62 (a) What is the significance of the clinical picture seen on the lower canine illustrated in *Figure 53*?
(b) What treatment would you advise?

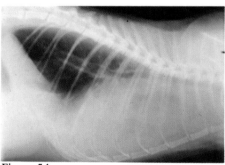

Figure 54

63 An 18-month-old male neutered Siamese cat has been showing tachypnoea for 6–8 weeks, especially following exertion. Within the last few weeks he has started to bring back some food soon after eating and is losing weight. Mucous membranes were pale but not cyanotic. On auscultation all chest sounds were very muffled and the ventral half of the chest was dull on both sides.
(a) A lateral radiograph of the chest is made (*Figure 54*). What is your diagnosis?
(b) How may it be confirmed?

64 An inexperienced owner presents the sand snake (Psammophis sp.) illustrated in *Figure 55*, and complains that it has 'bad eyes'. What would you advise?

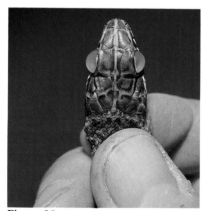

Figure 55

65   A 12-year-old entire male German shepherd dog was presented with a history of having collapsed the previous evening. The owner stated that the dog had appeared to become weak and had fallen over on his side. He was panting vigorously and seemed quite pale, but did not appear to be unconscious. After about half an hour he had gradually recovered, and by the following day he was almost his usual self. The owner admitted that this was the second time this had happened, the previous occasion having been some 10 days earlier. On examination the dog was bright, and in fairly good bodily condition. Chest auscultation was normal, with a normal heart rate and no murmurs. Capillary refill time was normal, although the mucous membranes appeared slightly pale. The abdomen felt rather soft, but no abnormal masses were palpable and no pain was elicited. Routine biochemistry and haematology results are given in *Table 5*.

Table 5

Total protein	64g/l	(55–75)
Albumin	25g/l	(25–35)
Globulin	39g/l	(30–40)
Urea	3.9mmol/l	(2–8)
Creatinine	52μmol/l	(<120)
ALT	26iu/l	(<100)
ALP	132iu/l	(<300)
PCV	0.32	(0.35–0.60)
MCV	85fl	(65–80)
MCHC	33.6g/100 ml	(30–40)
Total white cell count	11.2×10^9/l	(5–14)
Adult neutrophils	6.5×10^9/l	(4–10)
Eosinophils	0.9×10^9/l	(<1)
Lymphocytes	3.2×10^9/l	(1–5)
Monocytes	0.6×10^9/l	(<0.5)

RBC picture was quite markedly regenerative and not hypochromic. No abnormal WBCs were seen and platelets were adequate.
(a) What is the probable reason for the collapse?
(b) Comment on the probable aetiology of the anaemia.
(c) What is the probable underlying lesion responsible for this?
(d) How would you investigate this possibility further?
(e) What is the prognosis?

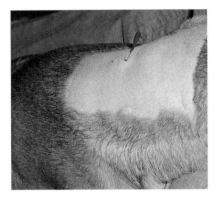

Figure 56

66 A young dog shows persistent discharging sinuses, one marked by a canula, on the dorsal aspect of the neck (*Figure 56*).
(a) What is the lesion?
(b) How should it be treated?
(c) What is the breed of the dog involved?

67 Anaesthesia is being maintained in a healthy dog with halothane in oxygen delivered from an accurate temperature-compensated vaporiser via a non-rebreathing circuit and endotracheal tube. What concentration of halothane would you expect to be giving this dog in each of the following cases to maintain a surgical level of anaesthesia?
(a) No premedication had been used and induction had been with halothane by mask.
(b) After premedication with acepromazine, anaesthesia had been induced with 8 mg/kg thiopentone.
(c) Induction of anaesthesia was with propofol (no premedication).

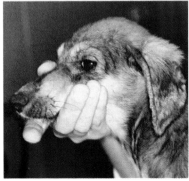

Figure 57

68 This young lurcher (*Figure 57*) has been extremely pruritic for 3 weeks following a visit to local woods. Lesions involve the elbows and hocks, and the owner reports a papular rash.
(a) What is your likely diagnosis?
(b) How would you confirm this diagnosis?
(c) If you fail to demonstrate a causal agent, how would you proceed?

69 (a) What is the injury depicted in *Figure 58*?
(b) What major structures have been destroyed?
(c) How would you treat this?

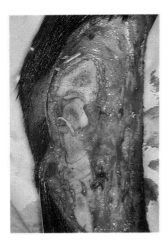

Figure 58

70 The Ionising Radiations Regulations 1985 stipulate certain requirements which a veterinary X-ray machine must fulfill. What are they?

71 *Figure 59* shows the plantar view of one hindfoot of a large New Zealand white rabbit.
(a) What is the probable diagnosis?
(b) How was the lesion caused?
(c) How would you treat it?

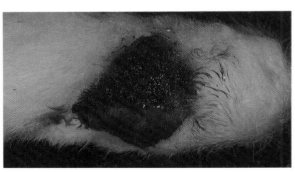

Figure 59

72 A group of three cats, 2 years, 18 months, and 5 months of age respectively, have all suffered from a bout of diarrhoea, with blood and mucus in the faeces, for 8 days. Fasting and kaolin/neomycin did not alleviate the problem, but metronidazole has dramatically stopped the clinical signs.
(a) Which of the following would you suspect?
    (i) Giardiasis.
    (ii) *Campylobacter jejuni.*
    (iii) Feline enteric coronavirus infection.
    (iv) *E. coli.*
    (v) Feline panleucopaenia (feline infectious enteritis).
(b) How would you confirm the diagnosis?
(c) What steps might you take to prevent reinfection?

73 A 5-year-old male cross-bred dog was presented with a complaint of persistent vomiting. The vomiting was sporadic and unrelated to eating, and there was no diarrhoea. On examination the dog appeared depressed, rectal temperature was 37.8 °C, and no masses or other abnormalities were palpable in the abdomen. The results of an initial biochemical investigation are given in *Table 6*, which were not considered significant. Over the next 3 weeks there was no appreciable clinical response to antibiotics or anti-emetics. No abnormality was seen on plain abdominal radiographs or a barium series. The vomiting remained sporadic but the dog grew progressively more depressed and an exploratory laparotomy was undertaken. No abnormality was found, apart from the unusual observation that although the dog's rectal temperature was slightly subnormal the temperature deep within the abdomen appeared to the surgeon to be abnormally high.

The results of a further biochemical investigation are given in *Table 7*. Haematology was unremarkable apart from a slight eosinophilia.

Table 6

Total protein	85g/l	(55–75)
Albumin	38g/l	(25–35)
Globulin	47g/l	(30–40)
Urea	12.9mmol/l	(2–8)
Creatinine	98μmol/l	(<120)
ALT	46iu/l	(<100)
ALP	102iu/l	(<300)

Table 7

Total protein	92g/l	(55–75)
Albumin	41g/l	(25–35)
Globulin	51g/l	(30–40)
Sodium	128mmol/l	(135–155)
Potassium	7.8mmol	(3.5–5.5)
Calcium	2.24mmol/l	(2.0–3.0)
Glucose	3.8mmol/l	(4–6)
Urea	24.6mmol/l	(2–8)
Creatinine	132μmol/l	(<120)

(a) What is your diagnosis and why is the age of the dog relevant to the diagnosis?
(b) What is the appropriate confirmatory test?
(c) What is the most appropriate emergency treatment for this situation?
(d) In what ways might the real diagnosis have been suspected from the initial biochemistry?
(e) How would you explain the apparent core hyperthermia with more peripheral hypothermia?

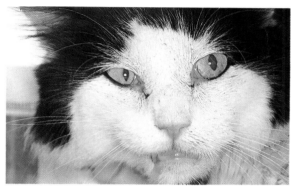

Figure 60

74 (a) What signs or neurological deficit are present in this cat (*Figure 60*)?
(b) What are the possible causes?
(c) Why are cats more susceptible than dogs to these changes?

75 The owner of the dog pictured here (*Figure 61*) requests orthodontic treatment to correct his animal's bite.
(a) What is your diagnosis?
(b) What treatment would you advise?

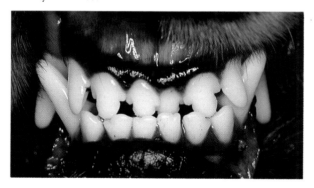

Figure 61

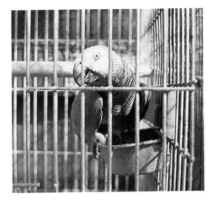

76 The African grey parrot (*Psittacus erithacus*) seen in *Figure 62* showed signs of stereotyped behaviour and dry lustre-less plumage. To what would you attribute these signs?

Figure 62

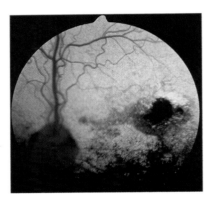

77 (a) Is the retina pictured in *Figure 63*, and belonging to a 6-year-old tricolour sheepdog normal?
(b) What are the distinguishing ophthalmoscopic features?

Figure 63

78 (a) How might you examine a bitch's cervix (*Figure 64*)?
(b) What information can be gained from this procedure?

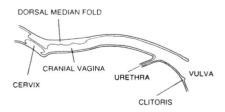

DORSAL MEDIAN FOLD

CRANIAL VAGINA

URETHRA

VULVA

CERVIX

CLITORIS

Figure 64

79 *Figure 65* shows a hand-reared kestrel (Falco tinnunculus), presented *in extremis*.
(a) What are the important clinical signs?
(b) How could this condition have been prevented?

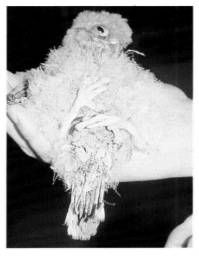

Figure 65

80 (a) What is the technical difference between these M-mode echocardiographic images (*Figures 66* and *67*), both of which were obtained from the right parasternal position in different dogs?
(b) What is the normal canine range for fractional shortening?
(c) How is this crude measurement of left ventricular contractility obtained?

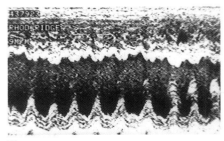

Figure 66

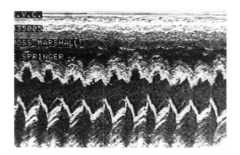

Figure 67

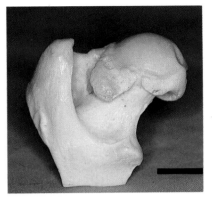

Figure 68

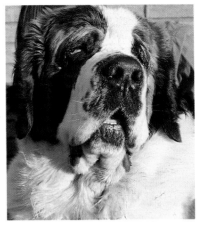

Figure 69

81 This femoral head (*Figure 68*) came from a young West Highland white terrier.
(a) What was the likely cause of the degenerative changes?
(b) What is the major vascular supply to the femoral head?
(c) List four surgical approaches to the hip joint and indicate which is most suitable for excision of the femoral head and neck.

82 A 3-year-old St. Bernard bitch (*Figure 69*) is presented with a history of increasing lethargy over a 5-month period. The bitch has put on some weight and her coat is poor. Her last season was 10 months ago.
(a) What is your tentative diagnosis?
(b) How might it be confirmed?

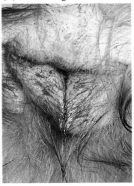

83 An otherwise healthy bitch is presented 3 weeks after an uncomplicated whelping with a scant mucosanginous vulval discharge (*Figure 70*).
(a) What is the probable cause of the condition?
(b) What is the prognosis?

Figure 70

84 The Amazon parrot (Amazona ochrocephala) seen in *Figure 71* had a swollen neck. When a needle was inserted, a gas (probably air) escaped. What are the differential diagnoses?

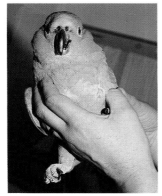

Figure 71

85 (a) What is an RPA?
(b) What role does an RPA play in a veterinary practice?

86 These feet (*Figure 72*), submitted for post-mortem examination, belonged to a parakeet which had been housed in an outside aviary.
(a) What are the lesions?
(b) How might they have been caused?

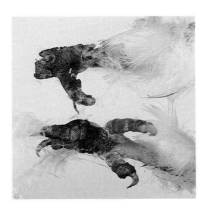

Figure 72

87 A 4-year-old rural male cat is presented with a number of crusty scabby lesions on its head and forelimbs. The lesions are about half a centimetre in diameter and some are purulent under the scab material. The cat has a mild pyrexia (39.4 °C) but is otherwise well.
(a) Which of the following is the most likely diagnosis?
    (i) Eosinophilic granuloma.
    (ii) Ringworm.
    (iii) Miliary eczema.
    (iv) Cowpox infection.
    (v) Feline leprosy.
(b) How might you confirm the diagnosis?
(c) How should the case be managed?

88 (a) What do you understand by the terms 'tranquilliser', 'sedative' and 'hypnotic'?
(b) Why is it important to know in which category a drug falls?

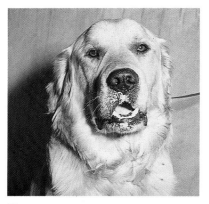

Figure 73

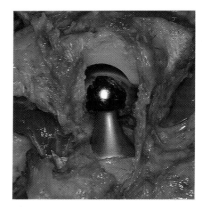

Figure 74

89 This 5-year-old retriever (*Figure 73*) has shown a sudden onset of dysphagia. Although it is enthusiastic to eat, it is unable to close its jaws and is therefore unable to retain food, fluid or even saliva within the mouth for effective deglutition.
(a) What is the likely cause?
(b) How would you confirm your diagnosis?
(c) What treatment would you recommend?

90 (a) What surgical procedure has been performed (*Figure 74*)?
(b) What are the indications for this surgery?
(c) What are the complications?

91 A 7-year-old neutered female Irish setter was presented with a complaint of blood in the urine intermittently over the previous week. On clinical examination the bitch was bright, but with a rectal temperature of 39.2 °C. There was a trace of blood at the entrance to the vulva and numerous petechial haemorrhages were seen on both the vulval and the oral mucous membranes.
(a) Which useful tests might be carried out if laboratory facilities are only accessible by post?
(b) Which useful tests might be carried out which can be done only in the presence of the patient?
Haematology results are given in *Table 8*.

Table 8

PCV	0.41	(0.35–0.60)
MCV	79fl	(65–80
MCHC	31.6g/100 ml	(30–40)
Total white cell count	9.4×10⁹/l	(5–14)
Adult neutrophils	5.8×10⁹/l	(4–10)
Eosinophils	0.3×10⁹/l	(<1)
Lymphocytes	2.9×10⁹/l	(1–5)
Monocytes	0.4×10⁹/l	(<0.5)

The RBC picture was moderately regenerative, no abnormal WBCs were seen and platelets were very scarce. Prothrombin time was 7 seconds (<12).
(c) What is the cause of the petechiation and haemorrhage?
(d) What is the probable diagnosis and how might this be confirmed?
(e) How would you treat this and what is the prognosis?

92 *Figure 75* shows a canary (Serinus canaria) with a subcutaneous raised swelling. What are the possible diagnoses?

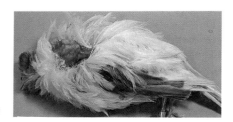

Figure 75

93 A 2-year-old fawn-and-tan Dobermann is presented with partial alopecia affecting the trunk.
(a) What are the features (*Figure 76*) revealed by skin scrapings?
(b) What is your diagnosis?
(c) Is there any reason why the owner should not breed from this dog?

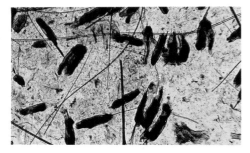

Figure 76

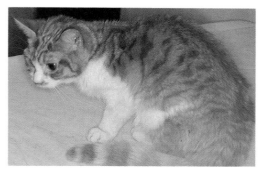

Figure 77

94 A 9-month-old domestic short-haired spayed female cat (*Figure 77*) is presented with a history of insidious onset of behavioural changes including ataxia and apparent disorientation. The cat has a mild pyrexia (39.4 °C) and does not appear to see normally. It has lost weight and is eating less well.
(a) What is the probable diagnosis?
(b) How might you confirm it?

95 (a) Is this retina (*Figure 78*), belonging to a 6-month-old liver and white English Springer spaniel, normal?
(b) What are the distinguishing ophthalmoscopic features?

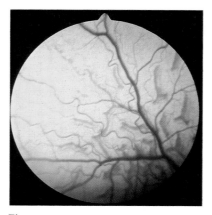

Figure 78

96 An adult male dog is presented with acute dysuria. Your attempts to pass a urethral catheter fail; the catheter tip meets a firm resistance at the caudal end of the os penis. Is this pathognomonic of urethral obstruction due to urolithiasis?

97 (a) What is the common name for the condition seen on the lower canines illustrated in *Figure 79*?
(b) Is it clinically important?
(c) Does it require treatment?

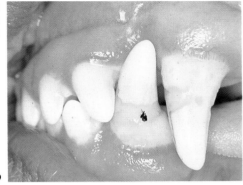

Figure 79

98 (a) Describe the pathology of the spine in *Figure 80*.
(b) What are the likely presenting signs of this condition?
(c) What complications have been reported, other than those related to the spine?

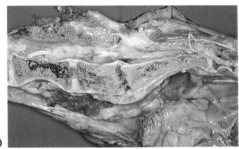

Figure 80

99 The cat in *Figure 81* is 13 years old and for the past 18 months has shown persistent ulceration of the rhinarium.
(a) What is the likely diagnosis?
(b) What treatment would you advise?

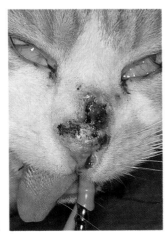

Figure 81

100 Describe the best method of performing cystography in the dog or cat in order to investigate suspected cystitis or bladder neoplasia.

101 Are triple phosphate or struvite calculi in the dog frequently associated with urinary tract infections with urease-producing organisms?

102 A 7-year-old Springer spaniel (a view of the ventral abdomen is illustrated in *Figure 82*) is presented with a history of weakness dating back over a month.
(a) What is the likely diagnosis?
(b) Are there any further historical features that would help in the diagnosis?
(c) What would account for the weakness?
(d) How would you manage this case?

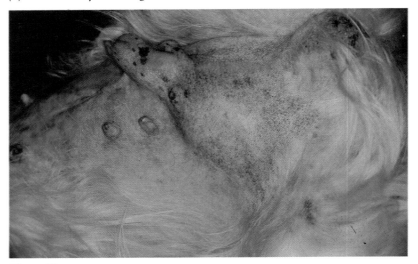

Figure 82

103 An 11-year-old cross-bred male dog is presented with weight loss and inappetence. Clinical examination reveals jaundice, which is confirmed on blood biochemistry. The total bilirubin is 25 mmol/l, of which 21 mmol/l is conjugated direct-acting bilirubin. The serum alkaline phosphatase is 1050 iu/l and the analine transferase is 340 iu/l. Blood urea is 6.5 mmol/l and albumin 23 g/l. Haematology reveals a slight neutrophilia and a mild non-regenerative anaemia.
(a) What type of jaundice is present?
(b) What is the most likely diagnosis?

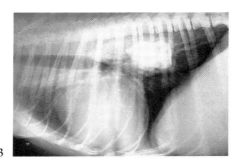

Figure 83

104 A dog was presented 48 hours after the acute onset of regurgitation. A lateral radiograph of the chest (*Figure 83*) reveals a radiodensity in the caudodorsal thorax.
(a) What is the most likely cause of this dog's regurgitation?
(b) What is the instrument in *Figure 84*?
(c) How may it be used in the management of this dog's condition?
(d) List some of the possible complications of this condition, including that demonstrated in *Figure 85*.

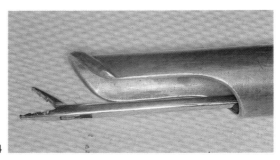

Figure 84

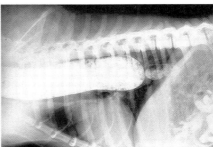

Figure 85

105 Acepromazine, xylazine and medetomidine are agents used to sedate and to premedicate cats and dogs.
(a) What effect does each of these drugs have on heart rate, arterial blood pressure and respiration?
(b) What other side-effects (of clinical importance) does each drug have?
(c) Which of these drugs can be antagonised?

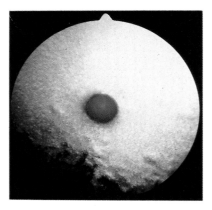

106 (a) Is this retina (*Figure 86*), which belongs to a 3-year-old black and white DSH cat, normal?
(b) What are the distinguishing ophthalmoscopic features?

Figure 86

107 This stifle (*Figure 87*) was swollen and crepitus was evident during manipulation of the joint. A mobile mass lateral to the tibial tuberosity was palpable.
(a) What is this mass?
(b) How would it appear radiographically?
(c) What is the treatment?

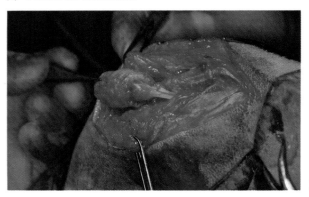

Figure 87

108 The guinea pig (Cavia porcellus) pictured in *Figure 88* shows photophobia and resists being handled.
(a) What is your diagnosis?
(b) What are the possible causes?

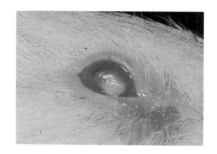

Figure 88

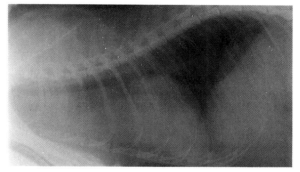

Figure 89

109 A 2-year-old cat is lethargic and coughing with tachycardia and a heart murmur on auscultation, and is referred because a heart condition is suspected. How would you interpret the two radiographs (*Figures 89* and *90*)?

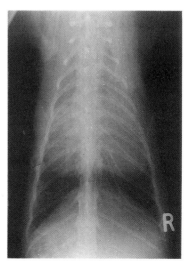

Figure 90

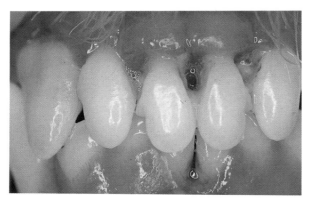

Figure 91

110 (a) What is the name of the disease evident in *Figure 91*?
(b) What organisms are usually present?
(c) What is the treatment?
(d) What is the long-term prognosis?

111 A 6-month-old Irish wolfhound is presented with a history of poor growth, poor appetite, and periods of profound lethargy and depression. Occasional episodes of pyrexia have responded to antibiotic therapy.
(a) What is your initial diagnosis?
(b) How might this be supported?

112 Describe the technique of non-manual restraint for radiographic hip dysplasia assessment in the dog.

113 A 7-year-old entire golden retriever bitch was presented with a complaint of poor appetite and marked polydipsia with nocturia. She had last been in season about 2 months earlier. On examination she was in fair bodily condition but appeared to have lost weight recently; she was rather dull and depressed, and had a rectal temperature of 39.2 °C. Mucous membranes were slightly injected. There was no vulval discharge and no abnormalities were palpable in the abdomen.
   A provisional diagnosis of closed pyometra was made and blood was collected for a total and differential white cell count. Results are given in *Table 9*.

Table 9

Total white cell count	$26.5 \times 10^9/l$	(5–14)
Band neutrophils	$6.6 \times 10^9/l$	(<1)
Adult neutrophils	$15.8 \times 10^9/l$	(4–10)
Eosinophils	$0.2 \times 10^9/l$	(<1)
Lymphocytes	$2.3 \times 10^9/l$	(1–5)
Monocytes	$1.6 \times 10^9/l$	(<0.5)

(a) How conclusive do you consider the diagnosis of pyometra is on the information given?
(b) What other differential diagnoses would you consider?
(c) What further tests would you advise?
A laparotomy was performed and the genital tract was found to be normal. A further blood sample was collected for biochemical tests and the results are given in *Table 10*.

Table 10

Total protein	78g/l	(55–75)
Albumin	25g/l	(25–35)
Globulin	53g/l	(30–40)
Calcium	2.34mmol	(2.0–3.0)
Urea	7.8mmol/l	(2–8)
Creatinine	102μmol/l	(<120)
Glucose	23.6mmol/l	(4–6)
Cholesterol	10.8mmol/l	(2.5–7.5)
ALT	121iu/l	(<100)
ALP	1645iu/l	(<300)

(d) What is your diagnosis?
(e) What is the reason for the neutrophilia and monocytosis?
(f) Why is this condition likely to occur in a bitch a few weeks after a season?
(g) What would be your initial approach to treatment?

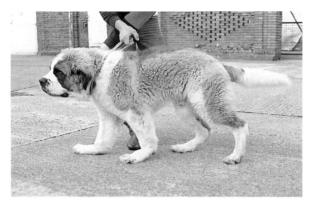

Figure 92

114 (a) What forelimb problem does this puppy have (*Figure 92*)?
(b) What is the cause?
(c) What is the treatment?

115 Match the patients below to the causes of obstructive dyspnoea on the basis of the known breed, age and sex tendencies. Select two dogs for each disorder. (Diagnosis should be based on breed, age and sex predisposition.)

Conditions
1 Nasal neoplasia
2 Soft palate hyperplasia
3 Laryngeal paralysis
4 Stenotic nares
5 Tracheal collapse
6 Glosso-epiglottic entrapment.

Patients
A 4-year-old Yorkshire terrier
B 11-year-old male labrador
C 2-year-old Border collie
D 18-month-old English bulldog
E 2-year-old Chow-chow
F 9-year-old female Afghan hound
G 6-year-old Papillon
H 4-year-old Border terrier
J 2-year-old English bull terrier.

116 A 12-year-old spayed Labrador bitch was presented with a complaint that two discrete masses, situated over the left lateral rib cage where they had been evident for some time, appeared to be enlarging. On examination these masses had the gross appearance of benign lipomas, with no features suggestive of recent enlargement. Subsequent discussion with a view to possible surgical intervention revealed that the bitch had become markedly polydipsic over the previous few weeks. Results of the initial biochemical investigation are given in *Table 11*.

Table 11

Total protein	64g/l	(55–75)
Albumin	26g/l	(25–35)
Globulin	38g/l	(30–40)
Calcium	4.23mmol/l	(2.0–3.0)
Urea	17.6mmol/l	(2–8)
Creatinine	232µmol/l	(<120)
Glucose	4.3mmol/l	(4–6)
Cholesterol	6.9mmol/l	(2.5–7.5)
ALT	83iu/l	(<100)
ALP	289iu/l	(<300)

Urine specific gravity was 1.003, otherwise urine NAD. Haematology was unremarkable.
(a) What do these results indicate?
(b) What is the probable diagnosis?
(c) What further investigations should be carried out to establish the exact diagnosis?
(d) What is the pathology involved in the polydipsia and renal dysfunction?

117 (a) Is this retina (*Figure 93*), belonging to a 2-year-old sable Shetland sheepdog, normal?
(b) What are the distinguishing ophthalmoscopic features?

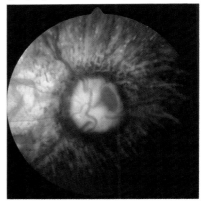

Figure 93

118 (a) What anticholinergic agents are commonly used for premedication of cats and dogs?
(b) In which circumstances would you consider their use essential?

119 Which of the following agents may be associated with kennel cough in dogs?
(a) Canine adenovirus 1.
(b) Canine adenovirus 2.
(c) Distemper.
(d) Canine coronavirus.
(e) Bordetella bronchiseptica.
(f) Parainfluenza III virus.
(g) Canine parvovirus.

120 A middle-aged male DSH cat has dyspnoea due to pleural effusion. The lateral chest radiograph (*Figure 94*) is repeated after drainage of the thoracic fluid.
(a) What abnormalities are present?
(b) What is the likely diagnosis?
(c) What therapy would you give?

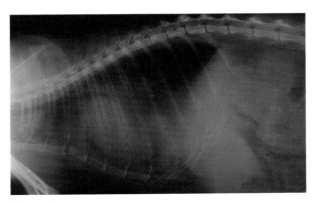

Figure 94

121 Can ureteral ectopia in the dog be diagnosed by performing a laporotomy and visualising the ureters as they by-pass the bladder?

122 An 8-year-old entire male English Setter dog was presented as suffering from 'fits'. The dog was never observed having a fit by the veterinary surgeon, but the owners described him as becoming wobbly on his legs and disoriented, before collapsing into lateral recumbency with tremors, leg paddling and jaw champing. These episodes had occurred with increasing severity over the preceding 10 days, usually in the afternoon. Clinical examination was unremarkable apart from the fact that the dog was slightly overweight.
(a) List your three main differential diagnoses.
(b) Which laboratory tests would you consider most important in this case?

Clinical biochemistry results are given in *Table 12*.

Table 12

Total protein	71g/l	(55–75)
Albumin	32g/l	(25–35)
Globulin	39g/l	(30–40)
Calcium	2.33mmol/l	(2.0–3.0)
Urea	4.6mmol/l	(2–8)
Creatinine	67μmol/l	(<120)
Glucose	1.8mmol/l	(4–6)
ALT	96iu/l	(<100)
ALP	204iu/l	(<300)

Haematology was unremarkable, with a normal PCV (0.48).
(c) What is the probable diagnosis?
(d) Which further test would you carry out to confirm this, and what is the full information necessary to interpret the result?

123 What are the advantages of rare-earth intensifying screens?

124 *Figure 95* shows an egg of a cock-atiel (Nymphicus hollandicus), labelled with a pencil prior to laboratory examination.
(a) What do you notice about this egg?
(b) What is the relevance of what you see?

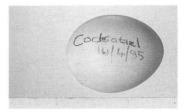

Figure 95

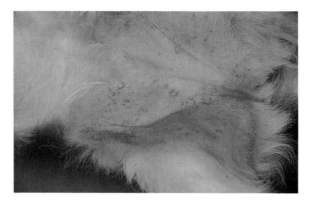

Figure 96

125 This 2-year-old bitch (*Figure 96*) is presented with a 1-month history of pruritus, especially ventrally.
(a) What primary lesions are likely to be present?
(b) What is the aetiology of these lesions?
(c) Name four underlying factors for this appearance.

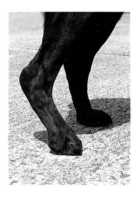

126 This dog (*Figure 97*) previously injured its Achilles tendon and has developed a crab-claw foot. There are no signs of a wound.
(a) What was the likely injury?
(b) Why does it produce a crab-claw foot?
(c) How would you treat this?

Figure 97

127 You are presented with a 5-year-old bitch, 4 weeks after her last oestrus. The animal is polydipsic, polyuric, and exhibits exercise intolerance with inspiratory noise. Its skin appears excessively thin, especially over the dog's head.
(a) What are the differential diagnoses for this condition?
(b) How may it be investigated and treated?

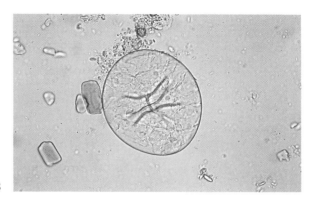

Figure 98

128 *Figure 98* shows a parasite found in the faeces of a goshawk (Accipiter gentilis).
(a) What is it?
(b) How would you control the parasite?

129 This puppy (*Figure 99*) has a rigid hind limb due to a polyneuropathy.
(a) Name two possible parasitic causes.
(b) How might the causes be differentiated?
(c) What is the treatment for both causes?

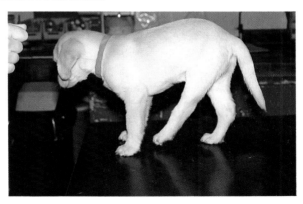

Figure 99

130 (a) By what routes may ketamine be administered to the cat?
(b) Ketamine is contra-indicated for use alone in the dog – why?
(c) With what drugs is ketamine best combined to reduce the problems?

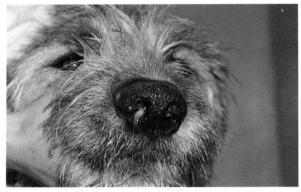

Figure 100

131 The patient pictured in *Figure 100* is a 6-year-old Irish wolfhound which has shown a purulent right unilateral nasal discharge for 3 months.
(a) List the possible causes.
(b) Specify the procedures which would be helpful towards a definitive diagnosis.

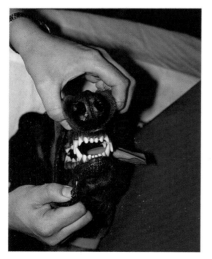

132 This Dobermann pinscher (*Figure 101*) is unable to open its jaws.
(a) What is the likely diagnosis?
(b) What is the likely pathology?
(c) What is the aetiology?

Figure 101

133 Is the radiographic finding of a caudally positioned bladder neck in a spayed incontinent bitch diagnostic of urethral sphincter mechanism incompetence?

134 *Figure 102* shows the plantar surface of a foot of a falcon (Falco sp.).
(a) What is this condition?
(b) How can it be treated?

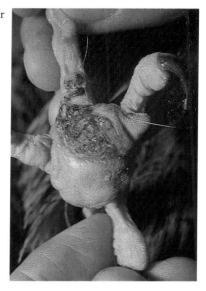

Figure 102

135 Which of the following statements about idiopathic canine epilepsy is/ are true?
(a) Fits generally occur when the dog is at rest.
(b) Fits are preceded by a prodromal period or 'aura'.
(c) Dogs with idiopathic epilepsy are normal between fits.
(d) Mysoline therapy should be stopped abruptly if the dog shows ataxia.
(e) Therapy, once started, has to be maintained for life.

136 Which of the following is the best surgical method of dealing with a dysuric male dog with urethral and vesical calculi?
(a) Immediate urethrotomy to remove the urethral calculi.
(b) Bladder drainage by cystocentesis followed by urethrotomy.
(c) Bladder drainage by cystocentesis, retrograde hydropropulsion to return the urethral calculi to the bladder and then cystotomy to remove the calculi.

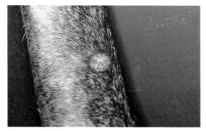

Figure 103

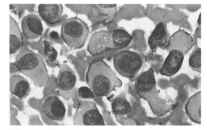

Figure 104

137 The mass seen in *Figure 103* has been present in this 3-year-old dog for a month; it appears to have been pruritic recently.
(a) Which two neoplasms would you consider in the differential diagnosis?
(b) Why must you differentiate between these?
(c) Which is represented in the cytology view (*Figure 104*)?

138 (a) When carrying out a pre-anaesthetic examination, what range of pulse rates would you consider normal in the dog and cat?
(b) What significance would tachycardia have for the subsequent anaesthetic?

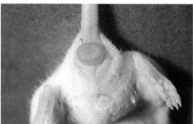

Figure 105

139 (a) What do you see on the mouse (Mus musculus) in *Figure 105*?
(b) How might it have occurred?

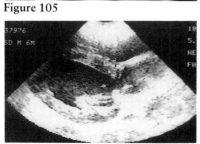

Figure 106

140 This ultrasound image of the left ventricular outflow tract (*Figure 106*) was obtained from the right parasternal position. The patient was a young German shepherd dog with a systolic murmur which was audible on both sides of the chest and at the thoracic inlet.
(a) What is your diagnosis?
(b) What is the prognosis?

141 What are the most common reasons for the failure of sedative drugs to be effective?

142 In which of the following is regurgitation a clinical feature?
(a) Myasthenia gravis.
(b) Pyloric stenosis.
(c) Feline dysautonomia.
(d) Mandibular neuropraxia.
(e) Persistent right aortic arch.
(f) Patent ductus arteriosis.

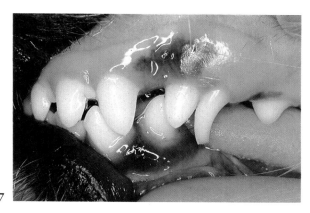

Figure 107

143 (a) What is the aetiology and sequel of the condition seen in *Figure 107*?
(b) What is the treatment of choice?

144 What is the length of pregnancy in the bitch?

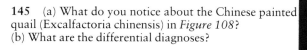

145 (a) What do you notice about the Chinese painted quail (Excalfactoria chinensis) in *Figure 108*?
(b) What are the differential diagnoses?

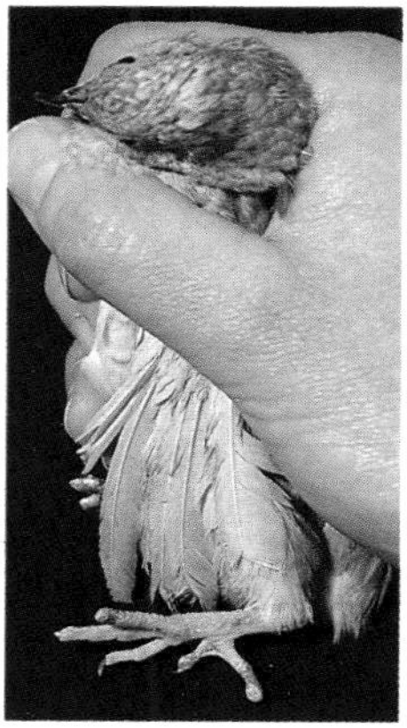

Figure 108

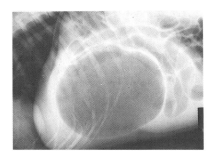

Figure 109

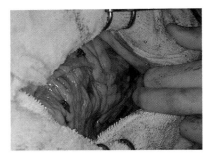

Figure 110

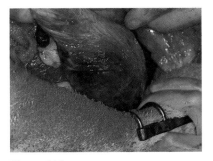

Figure 111

146 A dog was presented shortly after its evening meal with signs of dyspnoea, circulatory collapse, and a rapidly distending cranial abdomen. A right lateral radiograph of the abdomen, taken immediately on admission, is reproduced in *Figure 109*.

(a) What is the most likely cause of the dog's symptoms?

(b) What are your immediate priorities for management of this syndrome?

(c) What is the dog's acid/base status likely to be?

(d) At what point should a definitive surgical procedure be performed?

(e) What procedure should be performed in light of the appearance of the abdominal contents seen in *Figure 110*?

(f) What is the cause of the appearance of the gastric fundus in *Figure 111* and how should this case now be managed?

(g) What are the common longerterm complications of this syndrome?

147 Small animals with bladder rupture and uroperitoneum deteriorate rapidly and may die from the effects of which of the following – and why?
(a) Peritonitis.
(b) Acidosis.
(c) Alkalosis.
(d) Hyperkalaemia.
(e) Hypokalaemia.
(f) Uraemia.

148 *Figure 112* shows the firm swelling that has developed on the tongue of a young German shepherd dog.
(a) What is the likely nature of the condition?
(b) What treatment is necessary?

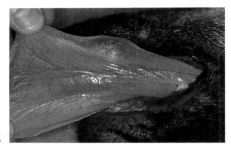

Figure 112

149 A 5-month-old entire Border collie bitch was presented with a complaint of slight polydipsia, occasional vomiting, and a general feeling on the owner's part that 'something wasn't right'. It was also mentioned that, although the bitch had been the largest of the litter when purchased, she was now the smallest of the group by some considerable margin. Apart from the small size of the puppy, which was readily apparent, clinical examination was entirely unremarkable. Heart rate was normal, with no murmur, mucous membranes were a healthy pink, and capillary refill time was less than 3 seconds. No provisional diagnosis could be made at this stage, and a blood sample was collected in the hope of further information being uncovered. Results are given in *Table 13*.

Table 13

Total protein	70g/l	(55–75)
Albumin	32g/l	(25–35)
Globulin	38g/l	(30–40)
Urea	1.7mmol/l	(2–8)
Creatinine	49μmol/l	(<120)
ALT	64iu/l	(<100)
ALP	510iu/l	(<300)

Haematology was entirely normal.
(a) What is the likely provisional diagnosis at this stage?
(b) What additional tests should be carried out to investigate this possibility further?
The low urea and raised ALP were considered to point to a provisional diagnosis of congenital porto-caval shunt. The dog was sent to the laboratory for a plasma ammonia test, and it was arranged that she be fed before setting out in order to obtain a post-prandial bile acid result as extra confirmation of the diagnosis. Further questioning of the owner at this time revealed that the puppy occasionally appeared disoriented, unable to find her way back if she wandered more than a few yards, and was in the habit of staring at blank walls for quite long periods. This type of behaviour is often seen in dogs with a porto-caval shunt. Results of the follow-up tests were: Ammonia, 165 μmol/l (<60); Bile acids (2h post-prandial), 0 μmol/l (<15).
(c) Comment on these results – are they consistent with the provisional diagnosis?
(d) Is there an alternative diagnosis which is consistent with all the facts of the case?

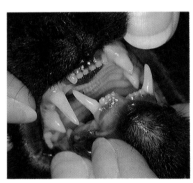

150 (a) What is this fracture (*Figure 113*)?
(b) What type of repair is indicated?
(c) What post-operative management is indicated?

Figure 113

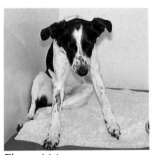

151 This dog (*Figure 114*) was hit by a car 45 minutes earlier. It is paraplegic and has hypertonic forelimbs and hypotonic hindlimbs.
(a) What neurological syndrome is evident?
(b) What type of cord damage is suggested?
(c) How would you attempt to localise the lesion clinically?

Figure 114

152 The haematology and biochemistry results in *Table 14* are obtained from a fasted 10-year-old Cairn terrier with a history of progressive alopecia, polyuria, polydipsia and weakness. The dog has received glucocorticoid therapy in the past for allergic skin disease.

Table 14

Total WBC	12,000mm^{-3}
Haematocrit	0.58
Differential WBC (%):	
Band neutrophils	4
Neutrophils	80
Lymphocytes	7
Monocytes	9
Eosinophils	0
Basophils	0
ALT	94u/l
Alk phos	78.3u/l
Cholesterol	8.5mmol/l
Glucose	7.9mmol/l

(a) What are the differential diagnoses?
(b) Which test can you use to differentiate between the two?
(c) What serious complication might be likely from these results?

153   (a) Is the retina (*Figure 115*) of this 5-year-old black Labrador retriever normal?
(b) What are the distinguishing ophthalmoscopic features?

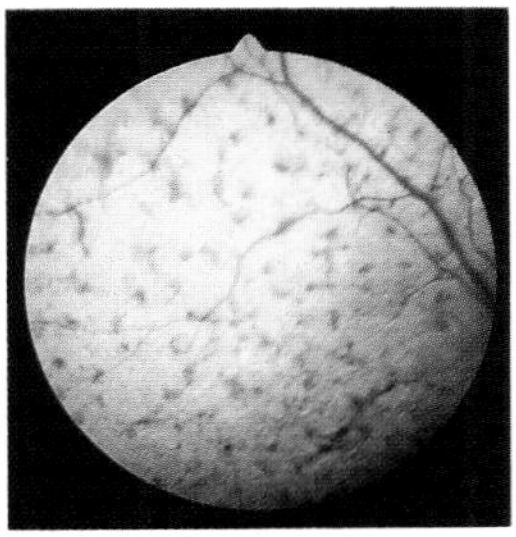

154   (a) What is scattered radiation?
(b) How can it be controlled?

Figure 115

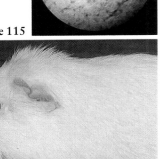

155   (a) Comment on this guinea pig (*Figure 116*) − It shows an important clinical feature.
(b) What are the possible diagnoses?

Figure 116

156 You have collected a semen sample from a previously fertile dog which has been unsuccessful at its last four matings. The whole ejaculate is clear and contains no sperm; the dog's testes are small and soft upon palpation. What is the likely diagnosis?

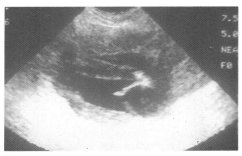

Figure 117

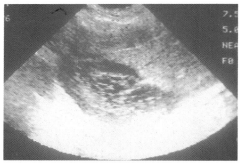

Figure 118

157 An 18-month-old Cavalier King Charles spaniel has severe dyspnoea and cyanosis on exercise, with a harsh systolic murmur, loudest well forward on the left side of the chest near the sternum. Two ultrasound images are shown (*Figure 117* and *118*), both obtained from the right parasternal position.
(a) What technique has been used to obtain the second image (*118*)?
(b) What is your diagnosis?

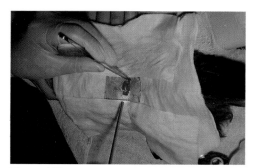

Figure 119

158 *Figure 119* shows exploratory laparotomy on a black kite (Milvus migrans).
(a) Why is the left side preferable to the right for this procedure?
(b) Why are birds good subjects for both laparotomy and laparoscopy?

159 Detrusor-urethral reflex dyssynergia in the dog:
(a) Is associated with a failure of urethral relaxation during micturition?
(b) Is associated with a failure of bladder contraction during micturition?
(c) May be voluntary or involuntary?
(d) Primarily results in urinary incontinence?
(e) Primarily results in dysuria?
(f) May respond to alpha-adrenergic blocking agents or diazepam?
(g) May respond to bethanechol?

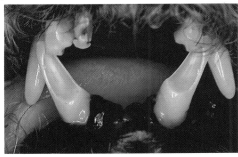

Figure 120

160 What is the aetiology of the condition seen on the lower canines in *Figure 120*?

161 What are the relative advantages and disadvantages of rebreathing and non-rebreathing circuits in veterinary anaesthesia?

162 *Figure 121* shows laparoscopic investigation of a ferret (Mustela putorius furo) with marked alopecia. List possible causes of this condition.

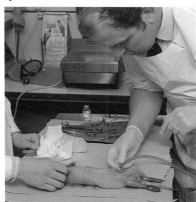

Figure 121

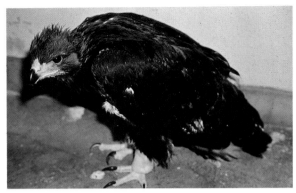

Figure 122

163 A golden eagle (*Aquila chrysaetos*), which showed weight loss, voice change and dyspnoea is seen in *Figure 122*. What are the differential diagnoses?

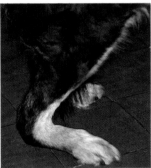

164 This collie (*Figure 123*) went acutely lame. There was no history of trauma.
(a) What is the likely diagnosis?
(b) What is the likely aetiology?
(c) How would you treat this?

Figure 123

165 A 7-month-old Siamese cat is small for its age and becomes dyspnoeic when handled and when it tries to play. Otherwise, it seems bright and eats well. A heart murmur is detected on auscultation. The most obvious clinical abnormality is illustrated in *Figure 124*. What is your diagnosis?

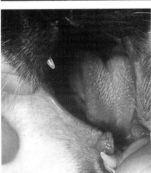

Figure 124

166 What physical properties affect the radiodensity of a substance?

167 Which of the following statements about *Leptospira icterohaemorrhagiae* is/are true?
(a) It is a water-borne infection, caught generally by dogs from swimming in contaminated pools.
(b) It is a major cause of renal failure in cats.
(c) It is diagnosed by culture of the organism from urine.
(d) It is a serious zoonoses.
(e) It is susceptible to penicillin and streptomycin.
(f) Protection requires annual vaccination.

168 The 8-year-old neutered female Cavalier King Charles spaniel seen in *Figure 125* has a chronic crusting lesion over the dorsum of the neck which has been getting progressively worse from some 4 months. The head tilt (*Figure 126*) has been present for 2 years and followed a middle-ear infection. The dog is generally bright but has become more lethargic and put on weight over the last 6 months. It eats well and is drinking more than previously.
(a) What is your tentative diagnosis?
(b) How might it be confirmed?

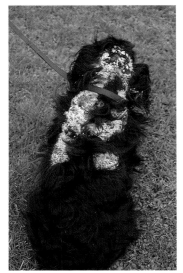

Figure 125

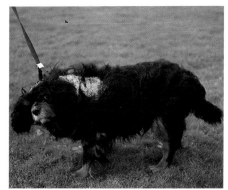

Figure 126

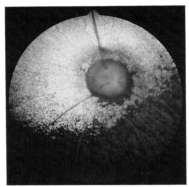

169 (a) Is the retina *(Figure 127)* of a 4-year-old blue roan cocker spaniel, normal?
(b) What are the distinguishing ophthalmoscopic features?

Figure 127

170 Which of the following conditions lead to asymmetrical prostatic enlargement and pain on palpation of the gland?
(a) Prostatic hyperplasia/metaplasia.
(b) Prostatitis.
(c) Prostatic abscessation.
(d) Prostatic cysts.
(e) Neoplasia of the prostate.
(f) Idiopathic prostatic haemorrhage.

171 (a) What is the differential diagnosis of the condition seen in the upper first incisors (*Figure 128*)?
(b) When would the condition be of significance?

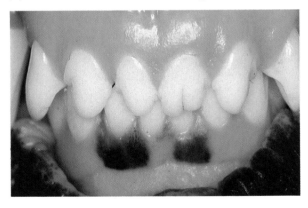

Figure 128

172 You have been asked to export some semen from a client's dog to the Republic of Ireland. How might you perform the practical aspects of this task?

173 The hedgehog (Erinaceus europaeus) seen in *Figure 129* has a skin lesion.
(a) What is a likely cause?
(b) How would you treat the lesion?

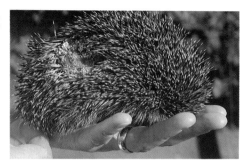

Figure 129

174 A clinical veterinary student has had this lesion (*Figure 130*) since nursing an injured hedgehog.
(a) What is the probable diagnosis?
(b) How might the diagnosis be confirmed?
(c) Which breed of dog is commonly infected from the same source?
(d) What is the prognosis for this condition in the dog?

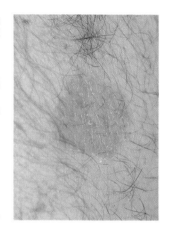

Figure 130

Figure 131

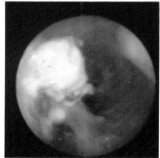

175 Anterior rhinoscopy of a 9-month-old cross-bred Doberman dog was performed to investigate a case of chronic unilateral nasal discharge. *Figure 131* shows cavitation within the nasal meati together with mycotic plaques on the mucosal surfaces. A positive serological result for *Aspergillus fumigatus* antibodies has been obtained. What is the treatment regime currently recommended for this condition?

176 What are the advantages and disadvantages of non-screen (envelope-wrapped) film?

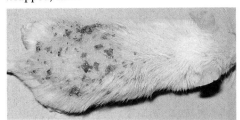

177 *Figure 132* shows one of a group of mice, of mixed sex, all of which show skin lesions. What are the possible diagnoses?

Figure 132

178 Which of the following statement(s) about tracheal collapse in dogs is/are true?
(a) It is seen primarily in young animals.
(b) Brachycephalic breeds are over-represented.
(c) It may present as a chronic honking cough.
(d) Excessive respiratory effort may precipitate a serious episode of collapse.
(e) Obesity is a predisposing factor in clinical disease.
(f) It can be diagnosed readily on plain radiographs.

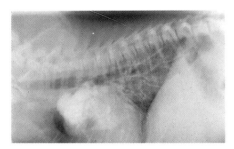

179 (a) What radiographic technique has been performed in *Figures 133* and *134*?
(b) Describe any abnormalities revealed.

Figure 133

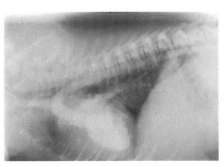

Figure 134

Figure 135

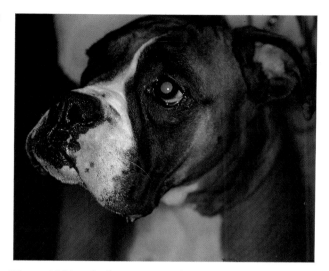

180 The dog in *Figure 135* has had non-seasonal pruritus since 2 years of age. There is a marked facio-pedal distribution and the condition responds to glucocorticoids.
(a) What is the likely diagnosis?
(b) Which test could you perform to help make this diagnosis?
(c) How might you manage this case?

181 Is the retina of the 1-year-old blue merle rough collie seen in *Figure 136*, normal?
(b) What are the distinguishing ophthalmoscopic features?

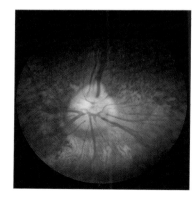

Figure 136

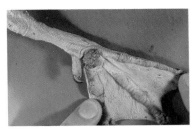

182 *Figure 137* shows a foot lesion on a mallard (Anas platyrhynchos).
(a) What was the likely cause?
(b) How should the lesion be treated?

Figure 137

183 The fractured maxillary alveolus seen in *Figure 138*, and belonging to a 5-month-old dog, is proving difficult to stabilise.
(a) What treatment would offer rigid immobilisation?
(b) What long-term complication may result from the trauma?

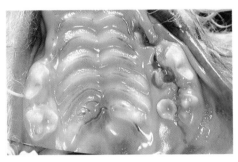

Figure 138

184 *Figure 139* illustrates a 2-year-old Boxer bitch with a 6-month history of weight loss, intermittent vomiting and variable inappetence. The dog frequently adopted the position shown and was said to lie 'stretched out'. She was bright and alert, and continued to be exercised well; the faeces were normally formed. What might be the cause of these signs?

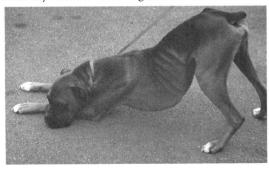

Figure 139

185 A young German shepherd dog has attempted to swallow a toy which has now become lodged in its pharynx (*Figure 140*). The owner rings for emergency advice because the dog is becoming cyanotic. It is unlikely that the dog will survive the journey to the veterinary hospital. What practical advise can you give to save this dog's life?

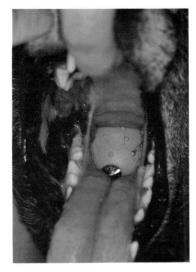

Figure 140

186 (a) Is the retina illustrated in *Figure 141*, and belonging to an 18-month-old yellow Labrador, normal?
(b) What are the distinguishing ophthalmoscopic features?

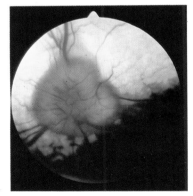

Figure 141

187 (a) What are the reasons for using neuromuscular blocking agents?
(b) What signs would lead you to suspect that a dog, given neuromuscular blocking agents, was inadequately anaesthetised?

188 What radiographic projections are likely to be most rewarding in the investigation of chronic nasal disease in the dog and cat?

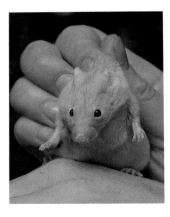

189 (a) What is unusual about this mouse (*Figure 142*)?
(b) What is the condition called?
(c) How would you confirm your diagnosis?

Figure 142

190 Which of the following statements about toxoplasma is/are true?
(a) The only definitive host for the organism is the cat.
(b) Once infected a cat continues to excrete oocysts for life.
(c) Infection is often asymptomatic in cats and people.
(d) Cats are the only source of infection for man.
(e) Pregnant women and immunosuppressed individuals are most at risk from toxoplasmosis.
(f) It is named after a small North African rodent, the gondi.

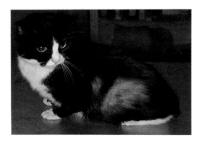

191 The 3-year-old cat in *Figure 143* was presented with symmetrical alopecia.
(a) How can you confirm that the cat is guilty of self-trauma?
(b) What are the three most likely differential diagnoses?
(c) Which haematological parameter might help in the diagnosis?

Figure 143

192 *Figure 144* is of a parasite from a captive barn owl (Tyto alba).
(a) What is it?
(b) How significant are such parasites on birds?

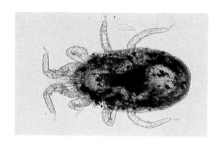

Figure 144

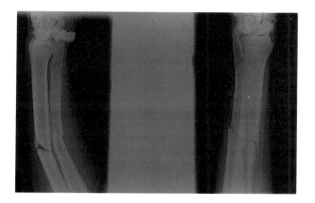

Figure 145

193 This radiograph (*Figure 145*) is supposed to demonstrate two views of a fractured radius/ulna in a dog.
(a) What film fault is evident?
(b) What might be the cause?

194 This dog (*Figure 146*) went acutely lame at exercise and is unable to extend its elbow. The proximal radius and ulna can be palpated lateral to the humeral condyles.
(a) What is the likely cause?
(b) What structures stabilise the elbow?
(c) How can elbow stability be assessed?

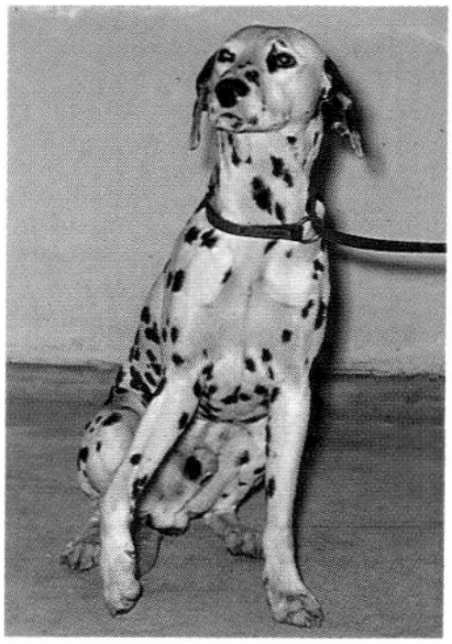

Figure 146

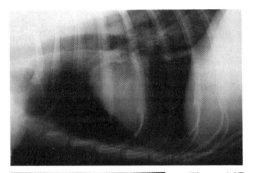

Figure 147

195 A 2-year-old female cross-bred dog was presented with a history of gradual onset of lethargy accompanied by occasional vomiting. The dog then rapidly became anorexic and dehydrated, with tachycardia and a weak pulse.

(a) How would you interpret the chest radiographs (*Figures 147* and *148*)?

(b) What biochemical tests would you ask to be performed urgently?

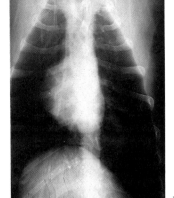

Figure 148

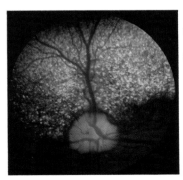

196 (a) Is this retina (*Figure 149*), belonging to a 1-year-old yellow Labrador, normal?
(b) What are the distinguishing ophthalmoscopic features?

Figure 149

197 A 7-year-old dog has hindlimb ataxia and hypermetric forelimbs (*Figure 150*).
(a) What is the likely diagnosis?
(b) What is the likely cause?
(c) How would you treat this condition?

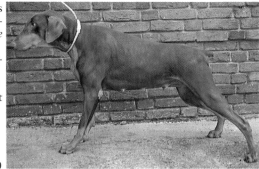

Figure 150

198 This dog (*Figure 151*) has an intra-articular tumour.
(a) What is the most likely cause?
(b) What radiographic changes are associated with this tumour?
(c) What is the prognosis?

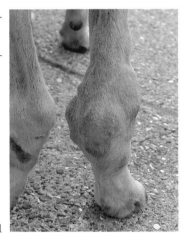

Figure 151

199 An 8-year-old domestic short-haired neutered male cat is presented with halitosis and reluctance to eat.
(a) What is this condition (see *Figure 152*)?
(b) What is the cause?
(c) How may it be treated?

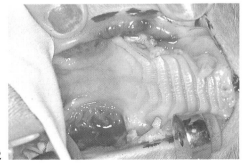

Figure 152

200 (a) In which animals is hypothermia during anaesthesia a serious problem?
(b) How would you attempt to prevent it?

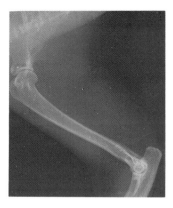

201 What film faults are evident on this radiograph (*Figure 153*) of a cat's humerus?

Figure 153

202 (a) Are plain radiographs useful in the diagnosis of tracheal collapse in the dog?
(b) Is fluoroscopic imaging of the trachea an accurate means to diagnose tracheal collapse?
(c) Is direct endoscopy under general anaesthetic the only consistently accurate technique to diagnose tracheal collapse?

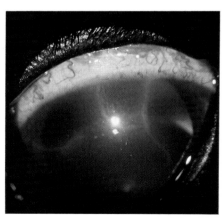

203 A 7-year-old Basset hound is suspected of blindness.
(a) What is your diagnosis (see *Figure 154*)?
(b) On what do you base this diagnosis?

Figure 154

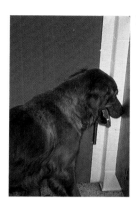

Figure 155

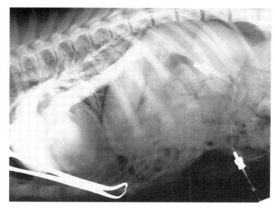

Figure 156

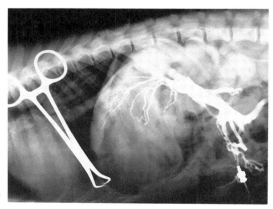

Figure 157

204 A 9-month-old Irish Setter (*Figure 155*) is presented in a comatose state 1 hour after having eaten a meal of chicken. The owners report that the dog is often dull, depressed, and aimlessly paces after food. It occasionally shows episodes of head pressing, and periodically it vomits and is polydipsic. Biochemical screening on admission reveals alkaline phosphatase, 245 iu/l; alanine transferase, 22 iu/l; urea, 2.1 mmol/l and creatine, 80 μmol/l.

(a) What is your provisional diagnosis and how would you manage the dog's neurological signs?

(b) What additional laboratory tests would you perform to confirm the diagnosis?

(c) Venography is performed via a jejunal vein (*Figure 156*). What is your interpretation of this radiograph?

(d) What surgical procedure should now be attempted and what parameter should be monitored during surgery?

(e) After surgery jejunal venography is repeated (*Figure 157*). Has surgery been successful?

(f) During the post-operative recovery period the dog begins to show sign of hypovolaemic shock. What is the most likely explanation for this complication and how should it be managed?

205 (a) The dog in *Figure 158* has a contracture of one of its shoulder muscles. Which one is it?

(b) What effect does this have on limb function?

(c) What are the likely histological changes?

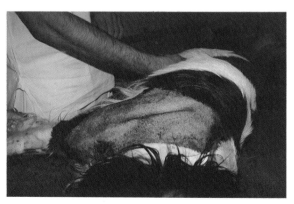

Figure 158

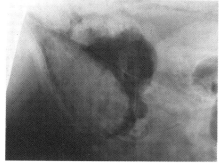

Figure 159

206 A 6-year-old entire Springer spaniel bitch is presented with a 3-day history of haematuria and increased frequency. On questioning the owner, it is learnt that the dog is drinking more than usual and has recently lost some weight. A plain lateral radiograph of the abdomen is made (*Figure 159*).
(a) What is your diagnosis?
(b) What further tests are indicated?

Figure 160

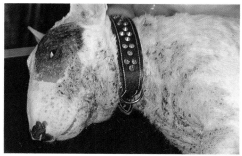

207 The 1-year-old English bull terrier pictured in *Figure 160* has had lesions progressing since 4 months of age. A skin biopsy section of the animal is shown in *Figure 161*.
(a) What is your diagnosis?
(b) Why was the diagnosis not made on skin scrapings?
(c) How would you manage this case?
(d) What is the prognosis?
(e) Is there any reason why the owner should not breed from this valuable dog?

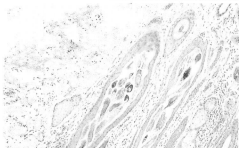

Figure 161

208 A 5-year-old entire female Cocker spaniel was presented with a persistent unilateral nose-bleed. The owner reported that the bitch was rather lethargic with an indifferent appetite, but there was no mention of vomiting, diarrhoea or polydipsia. The dog had been in season approximately 2 weeks earlier. On examination, she appeared moderately depressed. Rectal temperature was 39.9 °C, and the faeces adhering to the thermometer appeared black. In addition to the nose-bleed, there was some free blood around the opening of the vulva, and petechial and ecchymotic haemorrhages were seen on the gums, the vulval mucosa and several areas of the skin. Mucous membranes were moderately pale.

(a) What are the main differential diagnoses at this stage?

Table 15

PCV	0.26	(0.35–0.60)
MCV	67fl	(65–80)
MCHC	30.2g/100 ml	(30–40)
Total white cell count	3.7×10^9/l	(5–14)
Adult neutrophils	0.9×10^9/l	(4–10)
Eosinophils	0×10^9/l	(<1)
Lymphocytes	2.4×10^9/l	(1–5)
Monocytes	0.4×10^9/l	(<0.5)

Haematology results are given in *Table 15*. RBC picture was non-regenerative and slightly hypochromic, and no abnormal WBCs were seen. Platelets were very scarce. Prothrombin time was 9 seconds (<12).

(b) What is the cause of the bleeding problem?
(c) What is the actual diagnosis?
(d) How can this be confirmed?
(e) How might this be related to the recent oestrus?
(f) What is the prognosis?

209 A 5-year-old Labrador cross had shown signs of sneezing and left-sided epistaxis for 4 weeks. An intra-oral dorso-ventral radiograph of the nasal chambers was taken using non-screen film (*Figure 162*). What is your diagnosis?

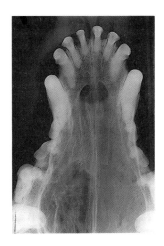

Figure 162

Figure 163

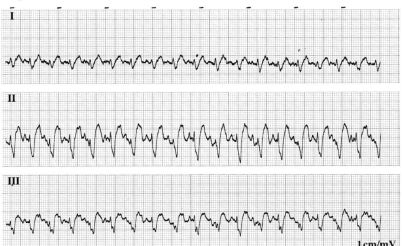

1 cm/mV

210 A 1-year-old St. Bernard dog was presented with dyspnoea and severe ascites which was resistant to treatment with diuretics. Facilities for ultrasound examination were not available, but an ECG and a chest X-ray were obtained (*Figures 163* and *164*, respectively). Another ECG was taken, several hours after treatment (*Figure 165*).
(a) What is your diagnosis?
(b) What abnormalities are present on the ECGs?

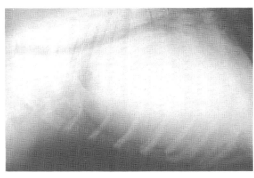

Figure 164

Figure 165

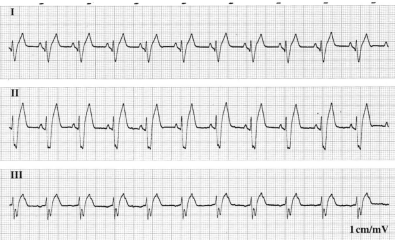

I

II

III

1 cm/mV

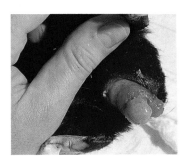

211 A female guinea pig is presented because the owner has noticed 'something red protruding from the vulva' (*Figure 166*).
(a) What is your diagnosis?
(b) How would you treat the condition?

Figure 166

Figure 167

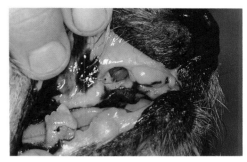

212 (a) What are the most common causes of an oro-nasal fistula (*Figure 167*)?
(b) What are the important factors in its treatment?

213 A 4½-year-old male Cavalier King Charles spaniel is presented with haematuria of 1 month's duration. Clinical and contrast radiographic investigations are unremarkable apart from the detection of slight dilatation of the left renal pelvis and proximal ureter, and vermiform filling defects in the bladder lumen during contrast cystography. Urine biochemistry, bacteriology and cytology reveal no abnormalities other than the presence of blood. During a laparotomy, the right ureter appears normal (*Figure 168*), but the left ureter is as shown in *Figure 169*.
(a) To what do you think this appearance may be due?
(b) What diagnoses might this suggest?
(c) What is the surgical treatment of these conditions?

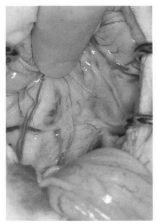

Figure 168

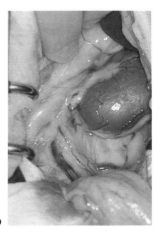

Figure 169

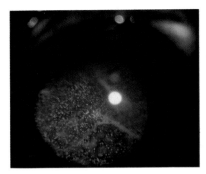

214 An 11-year-old golden retriever is presented on account of defective vision (*Figure 170*).
(a) What is your diagnosis?
(b) What other ocular conditions may be associated with this condition?

Figure 170

215 A 14-year-old male neutered long-haired cat (*Figure 171*) shows weight loss and diarrhoea. Appetite has increased, as has drinking, and the cat is said by the owner to be alert and active but 'short-tempered'. Initial blood test results are given in *Table 16*. Haematology was unremarkable.

Table 16

Total protein	84g/l	(60–80)
Albumin	26g/l	(25–35)
Globulin	58g/l	(25–40)
Calcium	2.14mmol/l	(2.0–3.0)
Urea	16.8mmol/l	(3–15)
Creatinine	172μmol/l	(<180)
Glucose	7.5mmol/l	(4–6)
Cholesterol	1.2mmol/l	(2.5–6.0)
ALT	156iu/l	(<100)
ALP	204iu/l	(<300)

(a) What is the differential diagnosis?
(b) What might you expect to find on clinical examination?
(c) How would you attempt to confirm the diagnosis?

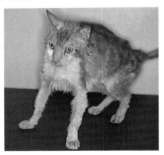

Figure 171

216 (a) Comment on the method being used for auscultation of the tortoise (Kinixys belliana) shown in *Figure 172*.
(b) For which diseases of chelonians is auscultation a useful clinical aid?

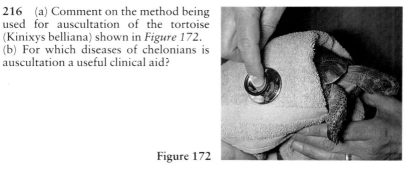

Figure 172

217 You are presented with a 4-month-old male dog with only one scrotal testis.
(a) What is your diagnosis?
(b) Which factors should you discuss with the owner?
(c) What are your recommendations?

218 *Figures 173* and *174* show the laryngoscopic findings in two dogs, both of which happened to be Irish Setters. Each had been subjected to partial laryngectomy surgery, in the one case, post-surgical progress was excellent, but in the other obstructive dyspnoea developed within 4 weeks.
(a) Why do you think the surgery was performed?
(b) What is the nature of the complication?

Figure 173

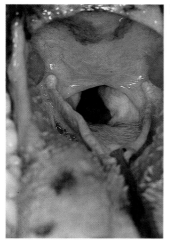

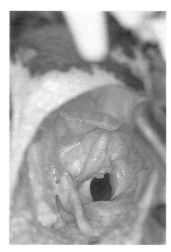

Figure 174

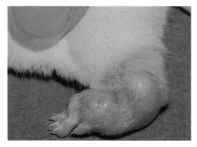

219 A number of breeding mice show swellings on their limbs (*Figure 175*).
(a) How would you investigate?
(b) What preventive measures might be advisable?

Figure 175

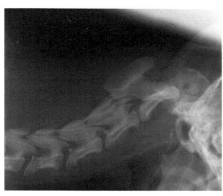

220 A 7-month-old Papillon has been presented as an emergency with acute neck pain and quadriplegia after falling off a chair. A lateral cervical radiograph is taken (*Figure 176*). What is your diagnosis?

Figure 176

221 This radiograph (*Figure 177*) shows a piranha (Serrasalmus nattereri).
(a) Comment on what you see.
(b) Is there any evidence of ill-health?

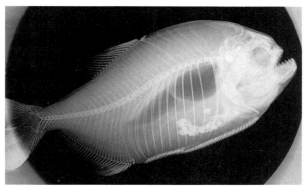

Figure 177

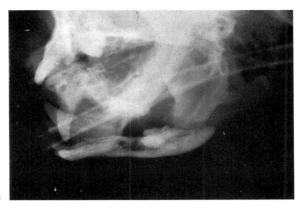

Figure 178

222 A middle-aged dog is presented with anorexia.
(a) What was the precipitating factor and what does the radiograph (*Figure 178*) reveal?
(b) What is the treatment and the prognosis?

223 This scaling alopecic lesion (*Figure 179*) on the pinna of a domestic short-hair cat has gradually worsened each summer for the last few years.
(a) What is the lesion?
(b) How might it be managed?
(c) Which serious complication may occur if treatment is unsuccessful?

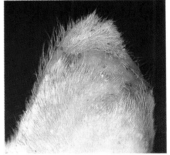

Figure 179

224 Advise is sought concerning a healthy 3-year-old dog which has recently begun urinating in the house and has a reduced appetite. Questioning reveals that the dog spends a lot of time sniffing the air in the garden, is restless at night, and urination is directed at vertical household structures. The dog's urine is normal on analysis.
(a) What is the likely cause of the problem?
(b) What treatment would you advise?

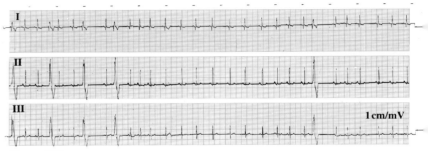

Figure 180

225 This ECG (*Figure 180*) was taken after a cardiac irregularity was identified on auscultation during a routine examination of a 7-year-old working Labrador dog. No loss of performance has been noticed.
(a) What treatment – if any – would you suggest?
(b) What would you advise for the future?

226 A 5-year-old entire male yellow Labrador was presented with a history of sudden-onset severe malaise and pyrexia. Clinical examination confirmed a rectal temperature of 40.3 °C, but no other significant abnormalities were seen. The dog appeared extremely depressed, however. Acute septicaemia was suspected and a blood sample was collected for haematology; the results are given in *Table 17*. *Figure 181* presents a representative section of the blood film.

Table 17

PCV	0.48	(0.35–0.60)
MCV	72fl	(65–80)
MCHC	33.6g/100 ml	(30–40)
Total white cell count	$286.0 \times 10^9/l$	(5–14)
Adult neutrophils	$0 \times 10^9/l$	(4–10)
Eosinophils	$0 \times 10^9/l$	(<1)
Lymphocytes	$286.0 \times 10^9/l$	(1–5)
Monocytes	$0 \times 10^9/l$	(<0.5)

(a) What is your diagnosis?
(b) Comment on the cytology of the blood film.
(c) What is the prognosis for a response to treatment?

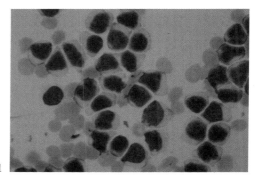

Figure 181

227 An adult cat is presented on account of a change in colour of one eye (*Figure 182*).
(a) What is your diagnosis?
(b) What clinical signs are present?
(c) What are the main possible causes?

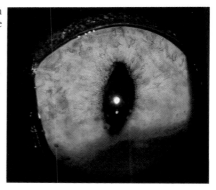

Figure 182

228 This dog (*Figure 183*) had an arthrotomy 3 weeks previously.
(a) What is the likely diagnosis?
(b) What radiographic signs are associated with this condition?
(c) What is the treatment?

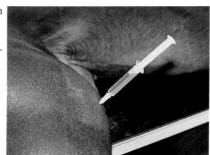

Figure 183

229 Two weeks after a routine ovariohysterectomy a bitch commences lactation.
(a) Has ovarian tissue been left in the bitch?
(b) How might you treat this problem?

230 (a) How would you decide if a cat required post-operative analgesia?
(b) What analgesics can be used in this species?

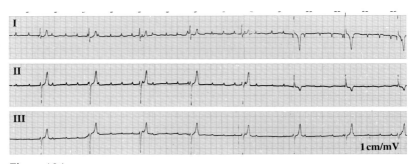

Figure 184

231 A 6-year-old Cavalier King Charles spaniel has had seven collapsing episodes/seizures in 1 day.
(a) What does the ECG show (*Figure 184*)?
(b) What treatment options are available?

232 This collie (*Figure 185*) suddenly became paraplegic while running in the garden 24 hours earlier. The condition is non-painful and non-progressive.
(a) What is the most likely cause?
(b) What is the treatment?
(c) What is the prognosis?

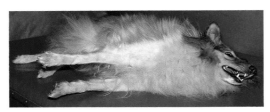

Figure 185

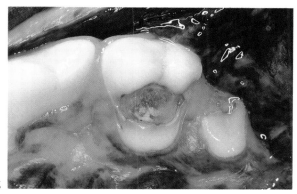

Figure 186

233 (a) What factors contribute to the condition illustrated in *Figure 186*?
(b) What are the treatment options?

234 The owners of a 5-year-old Rottweiler have noticed this pigmentary change (*Figure 187*) over a 6-month period.
(a) What is your diagnosis?
(b) Which three inflammatory conditions are associated with depigmentation?

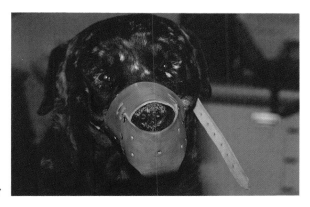

Figure 187

235 A 4-year-old entire female Springer spaniel was presented with a history of progressive exercise intolerance and weakness occuring over the previous week. On examination the bitch was slightly dull, with a rectal temperature of 40.2 °C. Respiratory rate was 30/minute and heart rate 190/minute. There was a marked systolic murmur, and capillary refill time was impossible to establish due to the extreme pallor of the mucous membranes. There were no signs of external blood loss and no petechiation. Biochemistry and haematology results are given in *Table 18*. RBC picture was moderately regenerative and not hypochromic. No abnormal WBCs were seen and platelets were adequate.

Table 18

Total protein	77g/l	(55–75)
Albumin	33g/l	(25–35)
Globulin	44g/l	(30–40)
Urea	5.1mmol/l	(2–8)
Creatinine	36μmol/l	(<120)
Bilirubin	15μmol/l	(<7)
ALT	94iu/l	(<100)
ALP	203iu/l	(<300)
PCV	0.11	(0.35–0.60)
MCV	92fl	(65–80)
MCHC	33.3g/100 ml	(30–40)
Total white cell count	17.1×10^9/l	(5–14)
Band neutrophils	0.9×10^9/l	(<0.5)
Adult neutrophils	11.8×10^9/l	(4–10)
Eosinophils	0.6×10^9/l	(<1)
Lymphocytes	2.7×10^9/l	(1–5)
Monocytes	1.1×10^9/l	(<0.5)

(a) What is the aetiological classification of the anaemia in this case, and what is the probable diagnosis?
(b) Which test would you use to confirm this and how heavily would you rely on the result?
(c) How would you proceed with treatment in this case?
(d) What is the prognosis?

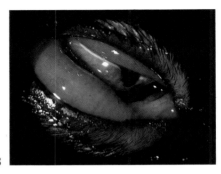

Figure 188

236 A kitten is presented with swelling of one eye and an accompanying mucopurulent discharge (*Figure 188*).
(a) What is your diagnosis?
(b) How would you investigate the case further?
(c) What would be your treatment of choice?

237 (a) What procedures would you employ to confirm a diagnosis of laryngeal paralysis in the dog?
(b) What surgical treatment is recommended for this condition and is it effective?

238 What methods can be used to reduce the pollution of the operating theatre by volatile anaesthetic vapours?

239 A 4-year-old miniature Schnauzer bitch is presented with a sudden onset of profuse diarrhoea containing fresh blood. The dog was normal a few hours ago but is now depressed and dehydrated; the temperature is normal. The dog is vaccinated.
(a) What is your diagnosis?
(b) How should the dog be managed?

240 The clawed frog (Xenopus sp.) pictured in *Figure 189*, showed lethargy and anorexia.
(a) What clue is there to the diagnosis?
(b) How would you treat the condition?

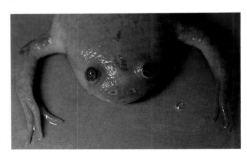

Figure 189

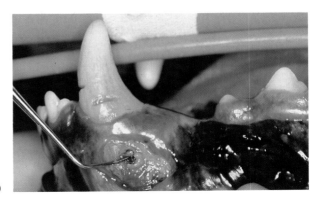

Figure 190

241 (a) What is the possible aetiology of the lesion seen in *Figure 190*?
(b) What treatment would you advise?

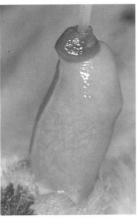

242 (a) What abnormality is present on this young male dog's penis (*Figure 191*)?
(b) What would be the major presenting sign?
(c) How would you treat the condition?

Figure 191

243 A breeder asks for a pre-mating bacterial swab to be taken from her bitch. What is the rationale for such action?

244 An 8-year-old Border collie bitch is presented as a second opinion with a history of exercise intolerance. She is obese with an irregular heart, but the pulse is strong and there is no murmur. Treatment thus far has been digoxin tablets prescribed by the bitch's usual veterinary surgeon.
(a) What abnormality is present on the ECG (*Figure 192*)?
(b) What would you do next?

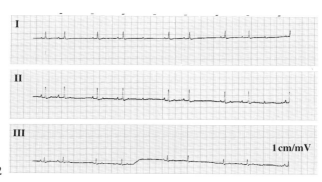

Figure 192

245 You are presented with a 2-year-old bitch that has not been in oestrus. The owners are keen to breed from her. Discuss your approach to this case.

246 (a) What is the aetiology of the labial ulceration seen in *Figure 193*?
(b) What treatment will give a predictable prognosis?

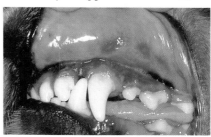

Figure 193

247 A 14-month-old male German shepherd dog is presented with intermittent right forelimb lameness of 8 weeks duration. Pain is detected on manipulation of the right elbow, and an X-ray is taken (*Figure 194*). What is your diagnosis?

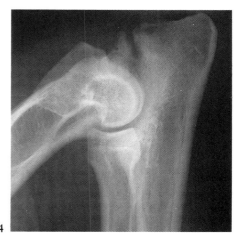

Figure 194

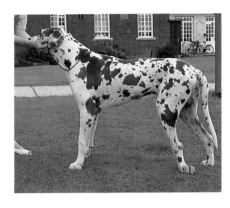

248   The dog in *Figure 195* is unable to extend its digits.
(a) Which nerve is involved?
(b) What are the likely sensory deficits?
(c) How might the diagnosis be confirmed?

Figure 195

249   A 9-year-old entire male Boxer was presented with inappetance, slight weight loss, and a history of progressive exercise intolerance over the previous 3–4 weeks. On examination the dog appeared slightly depressed and was a little underweight. Rectal temperature was normal, heart rate slightly raised and mucous membranes moderately pale. No abnormalities were noted on chest auscultation or abdominal palpation, although neoplasia was suspected in view of the dog's breed and age. Routine biochemistry and haematology results are given in *Table 19*. *Figure 196* shows a representative section of the blood film.

Table 19

Total protein	52g/l	(55–75)
Albumin	20g/l	(25–35)
Globulin	33g/l	(30–40)
Urea	9.6mmol/l	(2–8)
Creatinine	59μmol/l	(<120)
ALT	72iu/l	(<100)
ALP	96iu/l	(<300)
PCV	0.25	(0.35–0.60)
MCV	81fl	(65–80)
MCHC	29.4g/100 ml	(30–40)
Total white cell count	26.3×10^9/l	(5–14)
Band neutrophils	4.7×10^9/l	(<0.5)
Adult neutrophils	16.0×10^9/l	(4–10)
Eosinophils	0.6×10^9/l	(<1)
Lymphocytes	3.2×10^9/l	(1–5)
Monocytes	1.8×10^9/l	(<0.5)

(a) Comment on the red cell morphology and the other structures visible in *Figure 196*.
(b) Comment on the results – what is the apparent aetiological classification of the anaemia, and how closely can you describe the underlying lesion?
(c) How would you proceed with the further investigation of this case?

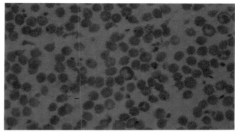

Figure 196

250 A 1-year-old guinea-pig is presented, having been looked after by neighbours during a family holiday.

(a) What is the lesion seen in *Figure 197*?
(b) Which organism is commonly implicated here?
(c) How might the neighbours have influenced the acquisition of this condition?

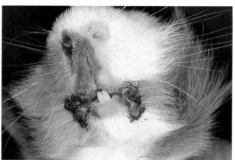

Figure 197

251 These feathers (*Figure 198*) were dropped by a vasa parrot (*Coracopsis vasa*). What is the significance of the differences in colour?

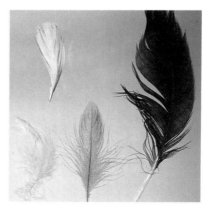

Figure 198

252 (a) Where can salivary cysts arise in the dog?
(b) What is the cause of these lesions?
(c) What treatment would you advise for their resolution?

253 A young cat is presented with bilateral ocular discharge, but examination of the bulbar conjunctiva reveals no evidence of inflammation (*Figure 199*).
(a) What is your diagnosis?
(b) On what do you base this diagnosis?

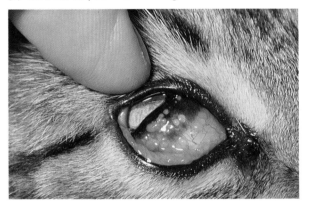

Figure 199

254 A dog was presented with dyspnoea shortly after being hit by a car; a lateral radiograph of its thorax is shown in *Figure 200*.
(a) What is the most likely cause of the dyspnoea?
(b) What are the immediate priorities for management?
(c) How should the condition be managed in the longer term?

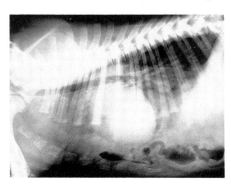

Figure 200

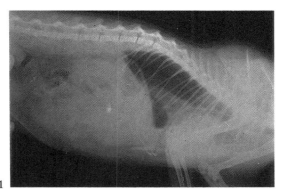

Figure 201

255 A chest radiograph of a very dyspnoeic cat is required to confirm diagnosis. *Figure 201* shows the radiograph subsequently obtained. What sedative or anaesthetic drugs would you use to restrain the cat:
(a) For the radiograph?
(b) For treatment?

256 (a) What is the name of the condition apparent in *Figure 202*?
(b) What has been suggested as a possible cause?
(c) What is the treatment?

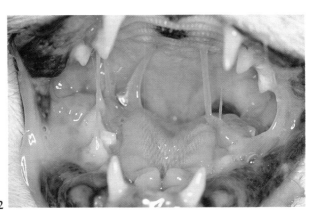

Figure 202

257 You examine a dog with signs of prostatomegaly, which is confirmed upon rectal palpation. Which other diagnostic steps may be taken to determine the cause of this problem?

258 A litter of 8-week-old pedigree long-haired cats are presented with a history of persistent 'gummy eyes' and ocular discharge for the past 4 weeks. There had been a mild nasal discharge at the beginning of the problem, but the kittens continue to feed. The queen is not affected and the colony is vaccinated against 'cat flu'.

(a) What is the likely cause of these signs?
(b) How would you treat the kittens?

259 A 7-year-old entire male domestic short-hair cat was presented with a bite abscess on his left shoulder. This sort of occurrence was not unusual with this cat, judging by the serrated condition of the ears and the moth-eaten appearance of the coat. On clinical examination he was occasionally fractious but seemed generally rather subdued. He was in fair bodily condition. Rectal temperature was 39.7 °C, abdominal palpation revealed no abnormalities but respiratory sounds were rather harsh. There was a slight nasal discharge. The teeth were quite severely encrusted with tartar and there was a moderate degree of gingivitis, but otherwise the mucous membranes appeared rather pale. The abscess burst during examination and was easily cleaned, but blood was collected for haematology because of the pallor and pyrexia. Results are given in *Table 20*. RBC picture was non-regenerative and normochromic, no abnormal WBCs were seen and platelets appeared adequate.

Table 20

PCV	0.21	(0.35–0.50)
MCV	47fl	(40–55)
MCHC	32.3g/100 ml	(30–40)
Total white cell count	4.5×10^9/l	(5–16)
Adult neutrophils	0.9×10^9/l	(4–14)
Eosinophils	0.2×10^9/l	(<1)
Lymphocytes	2.4×10^9/l	(1–5)
Monocytes	1.0×10^9/l	(<0.5)

(a) Comment on the results.
(b) What is your differential diagnosis?
(c) What further tests would you perform?
Further testing showed: FeLV to be negative and FIV to be positive.
(d) What would your advice be to the owner?

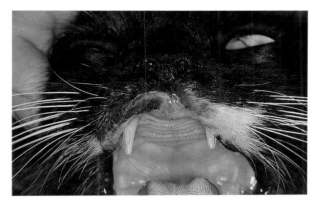

Figure 203

260 (a) What is the condition seen in the 8-year-old cat pictured in *Figure 203*?
(b) What are the treatment options and are they effective?

261 (a) What is the most common cause of stomatitis in a bird of prey, such as this young goshawk (*Figure 204*)?
(b) How is the infection acquired?

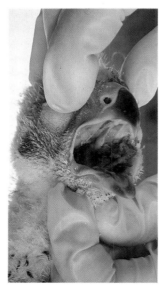

Figure 204

262 A breeder wishes to take a bitch to stud and is unwilling to leave the animal with the male; there are considerable distances to be travelled. How might you maximise the chances of conception in these circumstances?

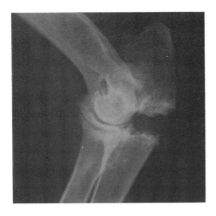

Figure 205

263 (a) What is the diagnosis in the case of *Figure 205*?
(b) What error was made in the repair of this fracture?
(c) What is the treatment?

264 A 10-month-old golden retriever bitch is examined because of exercise intolerance and bouts of apparent distress and panting. A Grade IV systolic murmur is detected in the mitral area, but the respiration is normal at the time of examination.
(a) What does the ECG show (*Figure 206*)?
(b) What might the dog be experiencing during the 'attacks'?
(c) What is this syndrome called?
(d) Can you suggest a suitable drug for treatment?

Figure 206

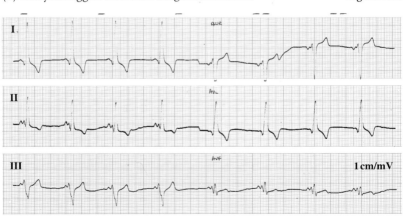

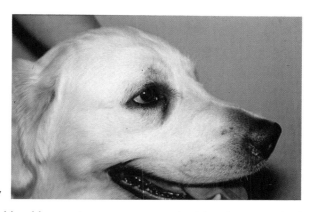

Figure 207

265 A 6-month-old golden retriever was presented with a brown-stained tear streak (*Figure 207*).
(a) What is your diagnosis?
(b) What are the possible causes?
(c) How would you investigate the case further?

266 *Figure 208* shows laparotomy findings in an adult female debilitated tortoise.
(a) What abnormalities are present?
(b) What structure are the two-shelled ova in, and can you explain how they got there?

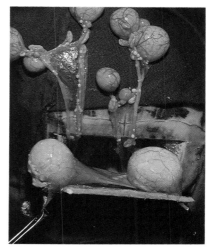

Figure 208

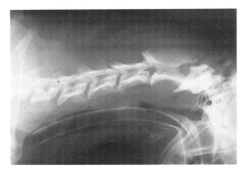

Figure 209

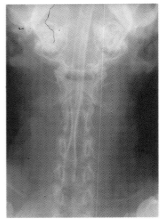

Figure 210

Figure 211

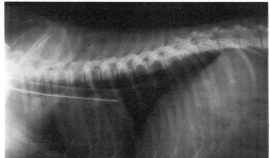

267 *Figures 209–212* demonstrate problems which have occurred with the use of endotracheal tubes. What has happened in each case, and what symptoms would the animal have shown? How could you prevent these problems?

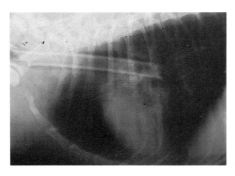

Figure 212

268 Lesions of which anatomical regions may result in the sign shown by this dog in *Figure 213*? This is the only clinical sign and the animal is otherwise well.

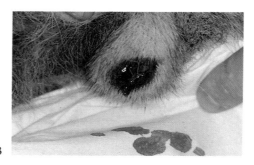

Figure 213

269 (a) Which of the following conditions may cause inflammatory responses in the integument of the ear canal of the dog and thereby underlie otitis externa?
(i) Atopy.
(ii) Dietary allergic dermatosis.
(iii) Contact hypersensitivity.
(iv) Seborrhoea.
(v) Pemphigus foliaceus.
(vi) Hypothyroidism.
(vii) Juvenile cellulitis.
(b) What are the dermatoses illustrated in *Figure 214* and *215*?

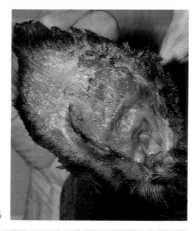

Figure 214

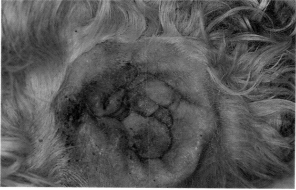

Figure 215

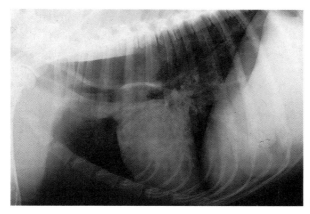

Figure 216

270   A 2-year-old Dobermann is presented with signs of depression, inappetance, weight loss and coughing of several weeks' duration. Occasional regurgitation of frothy material has been reported. Auscultation of the chest reveals increased lung sounds. A lateral chest radiograph is taken (*Figure 216*). What is your diagnosis?

271   (a) Which form of osteochondrosis is present in this elbow (*Figure 217*)?
(b) What surgical approach is required to remove the osteochondral fragment?
(c) List the other forms of osteochondrosis that occur in the elbow.

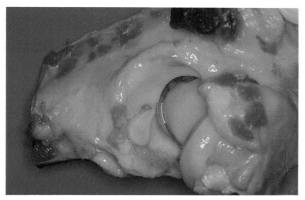

Figure 217

272   What special precautions do you need to take when you anaesthetise a bitch with pyometritis for ovarohysterectomy?

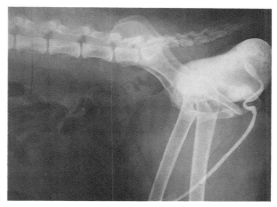

Figure 218

273 *Figure 218* shows positive-contrast retrograde urethrocystogram in a dysuric male dog.
(a) What is your diagnosis?
(b) What is the immediate management of this case?

274 A dog aged 10 months is presented with a recently traumatised canine tooth (*Figure 219*).
(a) What is your diagnosis?
(b) What is the treatment of choice and why?

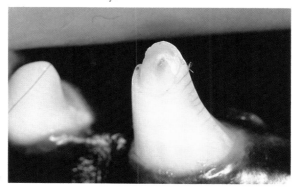

Figure 219

275 (a) What method of anaesthesia would you choose to anaesthetise (i) a cat, (ii) a bitch, for an elective caesarian section, where it is hoped to obtain live offspring?
(b) What special problems might you expect to encounter?

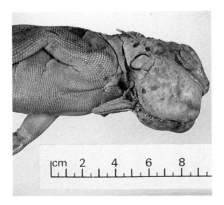

276 *Figure 220* shows an iguana with bilaterally symmetrical swellings on the lower jaw.
(a) What is the likely diagnosis?
(b) How would you confirm this?

Figure 220

277 A 1-year-old Springer spaniel is found to have a harsh systolic murmur, which is loudest on the left side of the chest quite far forward under the forelimb. The owner's concern follows the collapse of the dog while chasing a squirrel.
(a) What abnormalities are present on the ECG (*Figure 221*)?
(b) What would be your diagnosis?
(c) How could the diagnosis be confirmed?

Figure 221

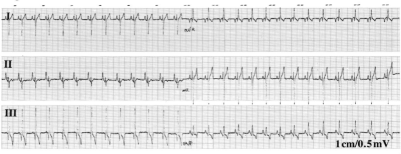

278 Which of the following factors are important in the management of chronic renal insufficiency in dogs?
(a) A plentiful supply of fluid.
(b) A high intake of non-meat protein.
(c) A low intake of high-quality protein.
(d) Additional salt in the diet.
(e) High phosphorus levels in the diet.
(f) Low phosphorus levels in the diet.
(g) Early management of intercurrent disease.

Figure 222

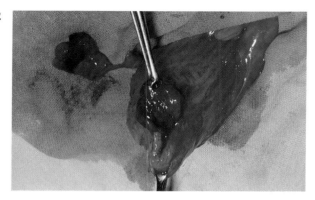

279 A male cat is presented with acute dysuria of 24 hours' duration associated with urethral obstruction by sabulous material. The obstruction is relieved by retrograde flushing, following which a urethral catheter can be passed without difficulty and normal urination is observed. A week later, however, the cat is presented with dysuria again. On this occasion there is no apparent obstruction to the passage of a urethral catheter but, once the bladder is emptied of urine, a doughy mass is palpable in the bladder. The cystotomy findings are shown in *Figure 222*. What do you consider has resulted in the second bout of dysuria?

280 A cat is presented for dysphagia. Examination of the oral cavity reveals these lesions (*Figure 223*), together with a history of recurrent vomition of fur.
(a) What are the lesions?
(b) How is this history suggestive of allergic skin disease?
(c) How can you manage the lesions?

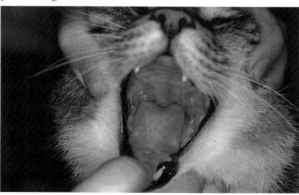

Figure 223

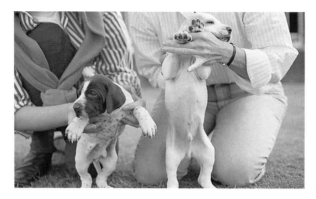

Figure 224

281 The puppy on the left in *Figure 224* has a genetic musculo-skeletal condition. It is poorly grown, has a flattened chest, and is developing a valgus deformity of its forelimbs.
(a) What is the likely diagnosis?
(b) What is its mode of inheritance?
(c) What other condition does it resemble radiographically?

282 A young Chow is presented with a wet eye.
(a) What is your diagnosis?
(b) What clinical signs are evident in *Figure 225*?
(c) What is the treatment?

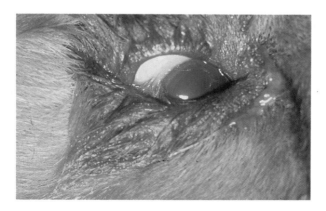

Figure 225

283 A 5-month-old entire male domestic short-hair kitten was presented with a history of inappetance, occasional diarrhoea, and poor growth rate. On examination the kitten was undersized and underweight, with a poor hair coat and a slightly 'pot-bellied' appearance. Mucous membranes were rather pale, rectal temperature was 39 °C, and there was evidence of recent diarrhoea. There were no cardiovascular or respiratory signs. The abdomen had a somewhat 'doughy' feel but no fluid could be obtained on paracentesis. A chronic viral illness was suspected and a range of biochemistry, haematology and serology tests carried out. Results are given in *Table 21*. RBC picture was non-regenerative and normochromic, no abnormal WBCs were seen, platelets were adequate.

Table 21

Total protein	102g/l	(60–80)
Albumin	21g/l	(25–35)
Globulin	81g/l	(25–40)
Urea	12.6mmol/l	(3–15)
Creatinine	142μmol/l	(<180)
Bilirubin	16μmol/l	(<7)
ALT	142iu/l	(<100)
ALP	403iu/l	(<300)
FeLV	Negative	
FIV	Negative	
PCV	0.20	(0.30–0.50)
MCV	46fl	(40–55)
MCHC	31.9g/100 ml	(30–40)
Total white cell count	22.4×10^9/l	(5–16)
Band neutrophils	0.3×10^9/l	(<0.5)
Adult neutrophils	16.9×10^9/l	(4–14)
Eosinophils	0.4×10^9/l	(<1.0)
Lymphocytes	3.6×10^9/l	(1–5)
Monocytes	1.2×10^9/l	(<0.5)

(a) To which diagnosis do these results point, and what are the most important findings in drawing this conclusion?

(b) What is the most important test to perform next?

An FIP antibody titre was carried out, and a result of 1:1280 was obtained.

(c) How conclusive do you feel the diagnosis of FIP to be, on the information available?

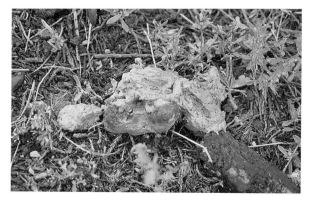

Figure 226

284 An 18-month-old German shepherd dog is presented with weight loss and a history of variable diarrhoea encompassing a period of 4 months. The dog is bright and alert and has an excellent appetite. It defecates in the waiting room; the results are illustrated in *Figure 226*.
(a) What is the probable diagnosis?
(b) How might it be confirmed?

285 (a) Diagnose the condition of the lower canine seen in *Figure 227*.
(b) Is any treatment necessary?

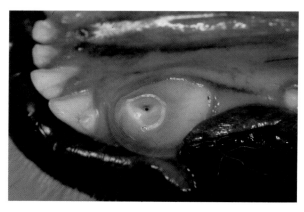

Figure 227

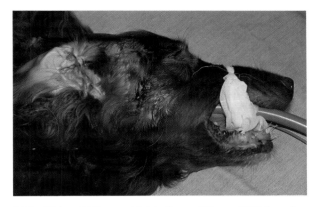

Figure 228

286 This middle-aged Irish Setter (*Figure 228*) has shown chronic suppurating sinuses on the side of the face. Several surgical foreign body searches have been performed in vain.
(a) What is the probable explanation for the complaint?
(b) How should it be treated?

287 *Figure 229* shows one of a number of parent-reared young cockatiels which stopped feeding and died.
(a) What was the likely cause of death?
(b) How would you confirm this?

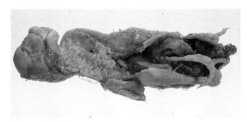

Figure 229

288 A 2½-year-old male neutered domestic short-haired cat (*Figure 230*) presented with a 10-day history of swelling of the limbs and ventral body wall. The cat is eating but has a reduced appetite and is not pyrexic.
(a) What is the probable diagnosis?
(b) How may it be confirmed?

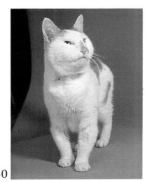

Figure 230

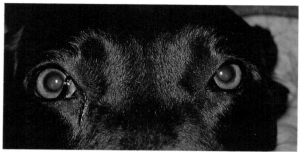

Figure 231

289 An 8-year-old Labrador retriever is presented on account of dissimilarity in the appearance of the two eyes (*Figure 231*).
(a) What is your diagnosis?
(b) What are the possible causes of this condition?
(c) What features depicted in *Figure 231* help you to reach your diagnosis?

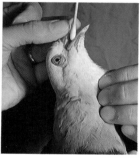

290 A throat swab is being taken from the pink pigeon (Columba mayeri), prior to its joining a breeding colony. Which potential pathogens pictured in *Figure 232*, might be recovered from the swab?

Figure 232

291 (a) Which ligament is involved in this avulsion fracture of the stifle (*Figure 233*)?
(b) What clinical signs might be associated with this fracture?
(c) What other structure is likely to be damaged?

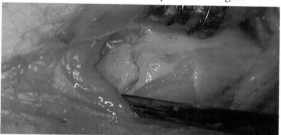

Figure 233

292 (a) What do you see in the buccal cavity of the python (Python sp.) in *Figure 234*?
(b) How would you confirm your diagnosis?
(c) What method of treatment would you follow?

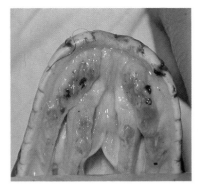

Figure 234

293 A 3-year-old Irish wolfhound is presented with weight loss, exercise intolerance and excessive panting.
(a) What does the ECG show (*Figure 235*)?
(b) What abnormalities are present on the chest X-ray (*Figure 236*)?

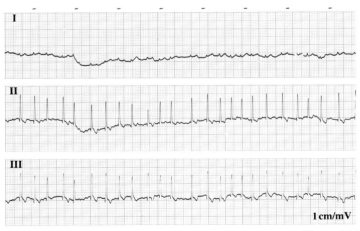

Figure 235

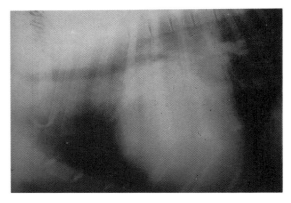

Figure 236

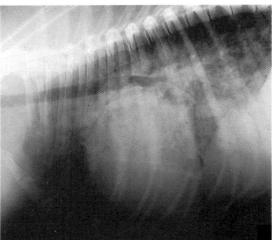

Figure 237

294 A 2-year-old male Dobermann has been seen as an emergency for acute-onset dyspnoea, with retching and gagging. The owner thinks that the dog may have swallowed a bone. Auscultation of the chest is difficult due to the dyspnoea but the heart rate is rapid and irregular. A lateral chest X-ray is taken (*Figure 237*). What is your diagnosis?

ANSWER ILLUSTRATIONS

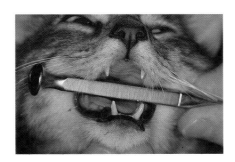

Figure 238

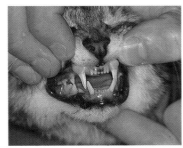

Figure 239

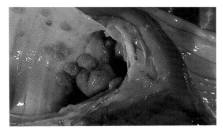

Figure 240

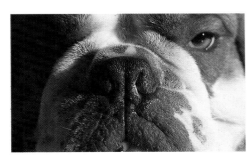

Figure 241

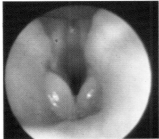

Figure 242

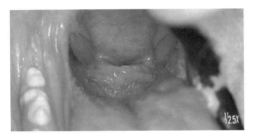

Figure 243

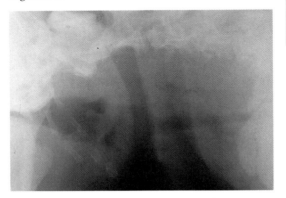

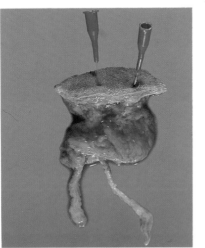

Figure 244

Figure 245

Figure 246

Figure 247

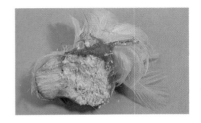

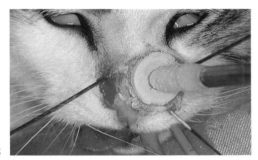

Figure 248

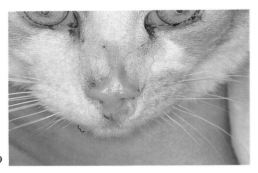

Figure 249

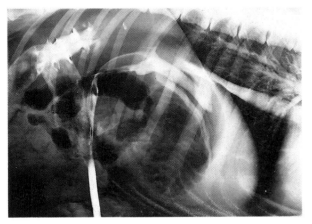

Figure 250

121

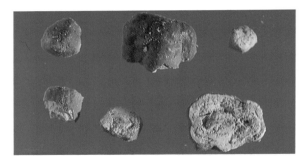

Figure 251

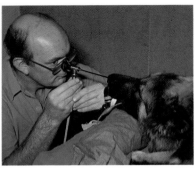

Figure 252

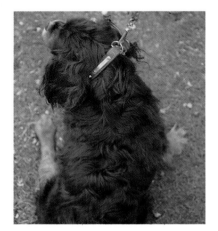

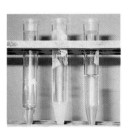

Figure 253

Figure 254

Figure 255

Figure 256

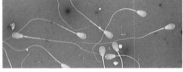

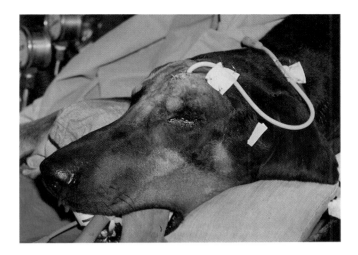

Figure 257

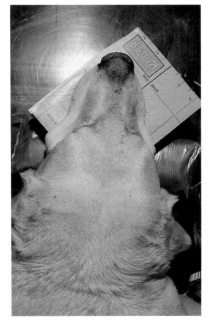

Figure 258

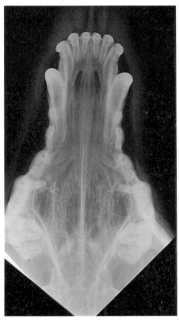

Figure 259

123

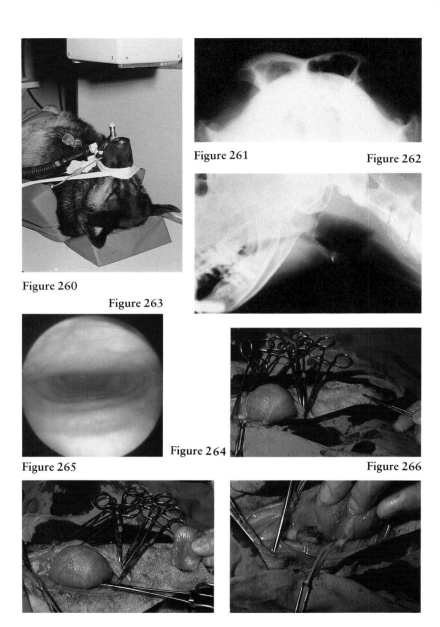

Figure 260

Figure 261

Figure 262

Figure 263

Figure 264

Figure 265

Figure 266

124

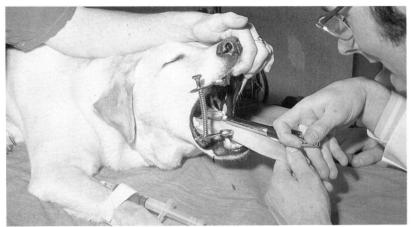

Figure 267

Figure 268

Figure 269

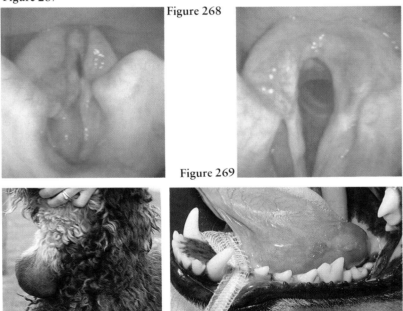

Figure 270

Figure 271

125

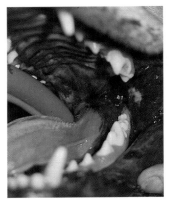

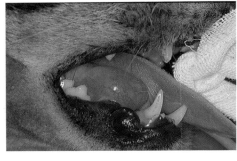

Figure 273

Figure 272

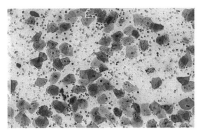

Figure 274

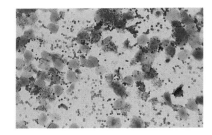

Figure 275

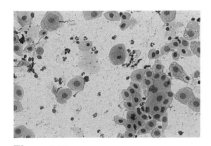

Figure 276

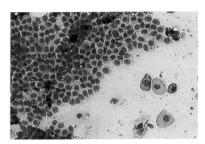

Figure 277

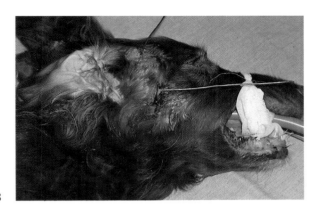

Figure 278

ANSWERS

*Illustrations for the Answers are given in the **Answer Illustrations Section**, pages 119–127.*

1 (a) Eosinophilic plaque and cowpox-like virus infection.
(b) Via skin biopsy or electron microscopy of crust material.
(c) A cowpox-like virus has been reported as a cause of skin, ophthalmic and systemic disease in man, contracted from cats.

2 (a) There is atrioventricular dissociation with multifocal ventricular ectopics (premature complexes) probably originating in the left ventricle. The QRS complexes are also wide (0.08 sec) with slurring of the ST segment. P waves are present in the middle of the trace but appear to 'migrate' into the QRS complexes; this is due to junctional tachycardia, when the ventricular rate is very slightly faster than the atrial rate.
(b) Digoxin toxicity, although deterioration can occur spontaneously. In this case, reduction of the digoxin dose restored sinus rhythm.

3 (a) A luxation of the right temporomandibular joint (TMJ) has been sustained. Note that the mandible is displaced towards the left side of the cat (the right in *Figure 3*).
(b) TMJ luxations in the dog and cat are usually induced by road traffic accidents and the mandibular condyle is displaced rostro-dorsally. Caudal displacement of the condyle is prevented by the post-glenoid process which supports the full width of the posterior aspect of the articular facet on the petrous temporal bone.
The radiographic diagnosis of TMJ luxations is surprisingly difficult partly because lateral-oblique projections are confused by superimposition of structures and partly because, on the more helpful whole skull ventro-dorsal view, the displacement at the affected TMJ is very subtle. Thus, diagnosis depends on the position of the jaw and the elimination of other bony injuries. Reduction of the luxation is generally achieved without difficulty under general anaesthesia. The mouth is closed by pressure at the chin while a fulcrum bar is placed transversly as far back in the mouth as possible (*Figure 238*). Confirmation of a successful reduction depends upon restoration of a symmetrical bite (*Figure 239*).

4 (a) A healing fracture of the distal radius with premature closure of the distal ulnar growth plate.

(b) Cranial bowing of the radius, lateral deviation of the distal limb, external rotation of the foot and reduced carpal flexion. Subluxation of the humero-ulnar joint may also develop, resulting in elbow pain and degenerative joint disease.

(c) Segmental ulnar ostectomy to remove the bowstring effect of the ulna, with transepiphyseal stapling of the cranio-medial aspect of the distal radial growth plate.

5 (i) **Make and type of X-ray machine.** It is not usually satisfactory to transfer an exposure chart from one machine to another, although it may provide an initial guide.

(ii) **Focal-film distance (FFD).** Whenever possible the FFD should be kept constant, since the intensity of the beam varies inversely according to the square of the distance (the **inverse square law**).

(iii) **Film-screen combination.** Screen film in combination with intensifying screens allows the use of much lower exposure factors than when direct-exposure film is employed. However, different types of both film and screen vary with regard to their speed. It is preferable, therefore, to use the same film-screen combination, otherwise a compensatory adjustment of the exposure factors will be required.

(iv) **Grid.** The use of a grid will always involve an increase in exposure, which can be worked out from the **grid factor**.

(v) **Processing.** The use of an exposure chart is absolutely dependent on an efficient and standardised processing technique.

(vi) **Thickness and nature of the area under investigation, and the presence or absence of any pathological changes within it.** Thus, an exposure chart should contain information on the area under investigation, the projection and the size of the patient.

(vii) **Kilovoltage (kV).** The kV control regulates the penetrating power of the X-ray beam. The use of too high kV will result in an overpenetrated 'flat' film that lacks contrast.

(viii) **Milliampere-seconds (mAs).** Milliamperage and time are considered together because of their close relationship. The mAs control is used to produce optimal density and detail on the radiograph. Time should be kept as short as possible to avoid movement blur, and thus the mA is usually set at its maximum.

6 (a) Keratoconjunctivitis sicca, or 'dry eye'.

(b) Chronic keratitis (vascularisation) with mucopurulent discharge sticking to the cornea and eyelid margins.

(c) Schirmer tear test.

7 The point of the ultrasonic tip must never be used for the scaling procedure as it would create irreversible scratches in the dentine and enamel, which would encourage a rapid build-up of plaque and calculus formation. Only the sides of the scaling tip should be used.

8 The radiographic changes are typical of hypervitaminosis A, associated with prolonged feeding of a diet high in uncooked liver. There is organised new bone bridging the joint, with some loss of overall bone density but no areas of lysis. These features differentiate the changes from those of bone neoplasia. Although typically described as an ankylosing cervical spondylopathy, hypervitaminosis A not infrequently presents as lameness due to exostoses around limb joints. There may also be new bone involving the lower spinal column but this may not be clinically obvious. A change to a balanced diet, not always easily achieved, leads to some improvement. Removal of new bone should be attempted only after some weeks on a normal diet.

9 (a) The main considerations in this case, initially, were a foreign body in the small intestine, acute necrotising pancreatitis, and renal failure.

(b) Radiography should not be omitted even though no foreign body was palpable, since the possibility of missing something on palpation can never be dismissed (and if no positive diagnosis had emerged from the blood results, contrast radiography would have had to have been attempted). The most important blood tests are amylase and lipase (to check for pancreatitis), urea and creatinine (to check for renal failure), and sodium and potassium (to help rationalise any subsequent fluid therapy), but virtually all of the tests listed gave useful results in this case.

(c) The diagnosis is clearly renal failure, as can be seen from the urea and creatinine results, and despite the apparently acute onset the condition is almost certainly chronic. The non-regenerative anaemia (evident in spite of the dehydration) indicates that the kidneys have been failing for some time, as it takes several weeks or even months for a deficiency of erythropoietin (produced by the kidneys) to manifest itself in clinical anaemia. In addition, the slight hypokalaemia (a result of the vomiting) suggests a non-acute renal failure, as acute renal failure with oliguria/anuria is more likely to produce hyperkalaemia. It is virtually certain that this dog had been polydipsic for some time before the onset of the current crisis, although, where an assessment of actual volume intake cannot be elucidated, this can be very difficult to prove, and it is not unusual for even severe polydipsia to be accepted as 'normal' by an owner if it has continued for a long time. Anorexia preceding the onset of the vomiting is another reasonable assumption which could not be verified in this case.

(d) Fairly marked signs of systemic infection in the white cell picture are quite common in this type of case, probably as a result of the gastritis and gingivitis. The raised amylase is an incidental finding due to the inability of the failing kidneys to excrete this enzyme, as would normally occur (lipase, too, is seen to be elevated in these cases from time to time). The important point here is that if, initially only amylase and a white cell count had been done, with pancreatitis as the main provisional diagnosis, a misleading diagnosis could easily have been reached.

(e) The prognosis is hopeless. When plasma creatinine concentration exceeds 700 µmol/l in chronic renal failure, prognosis is always poor. If the patient is reasonably bright and prepared to eat, it may be worth attempting intensive treatment, but when a dog is presented as ill as this one was, such attempts are ill-advised.

10 (a) A = Magill circuit, B = Lack circuit (co-axial adaptation of the Magill), Ca = Ayres T-piece, Cb = Jackson-Rees modification of the Ayres T-piece (i.e., the addition of an open-ended bag), and D = Modified Bain (a co-axial modification of the T-piece).

(b) To ensure no rebreathing, flow rates 1–1.25 times the animal's minute volume are used with the Magill and Lack circuits, and flows of twice the minute volume are used with the T-piece and Bain circuits.

(c) The T-piece (C) would be suitable for use in a cat, having a very low resistance, and dead space. The Bain (D) should also be suitable, theoretically, but the valve shown in *Figure 8* could give too much resistance for a cat. For the dog, the Magill, Lack or Bain circuit could be used, although higher gas flows would be required with the Bain.

11 (a) Perineal urethrostomy.

(b) One indication is permanently to by-pass a more distal, permanent urethral obstruction such as irreparable, extensive trauma; neoplasia (urethral or penile), associated with radical excision of the tumour; or urethral stricture.

Perineal urethrostomy is also sometimes used to remove calculi or allow instrumentation of the pelvic, prostatic urethra and bladder (e.g., urethrocystoscopy, lithotrypsy), but does not require creation of a permanent stoma.

Post-operative complications of perineal urethrostomy include haemorrhage from the corpus spongiosus, wound breakdown (possibly leading to subcutaneous urine leakage, resulting in necrosis), obstruction of the stoma by blood clots, stricture of the stoma, and recurring urinary tract infections.

12 (a) It is impossible to say how severely affected the bird is since, although there appears to be little on the plumage, substantial quantities of oil may have been ingested – perhaps during preening.
(b) Initial treatment should consist of nursing and administration of laxatives to hasten passage of any ingested oil. Further preening must be discouraged until the oil has been removed.

13 (a) One leg is thicker than the other.
(b) Possible diagnoses are a fracture, nutritional osteodystrophy, a haematoma, oedema, a reaction to an irritant injection, or infective osteitis. In this case the last of these was the correct diagnosis – and was confirmed by radiography.

14 Conceptuses can usually be imaged at 21–23 days of pregnancy. However, since the beginning of pregnancy cannot be easily defined, and because there is rarely any necessity for an early diagnosis of gestation in the bitch, scanning should not be routinely attempted at this time. By 28 days the conceptuses are bigger and a more accurate assessment of their numbers can be made. However, it is wrong to offer to predict how many pups are going to be born, first because resorption of some conceptuses does occur, and secondly because underestimates of the number of conceptuses are easily made, especially where large numbers are present (parts of the uterus can become hidden behind intestine).

As pregnancy progresses, individual pups lying close to the body wall can be detected in more detail, but estimates of numbers become progressively more inaccurate. In later pregnancy, foetal abnormalities may be detected and foetal viability can be confirmed by imaging the moving heart.

15 (a) Juvenile vaginitis. The cause is unknown and the condition is not associated with malaise. The discharge is composed mainly of vaginal epithelial cells but neutrophils may be present too.
(b) The discharge spontaneously resolves after the first oestrus and requires no treatment. Antibiotic therapy may produce a temporary response but is unnecessary and raises the owner's expectations of a cure.

16 (a) Gastric ulceration, possibly a manifestation of an enterotoxaemia.
(b) Rabbits, like rodents, can react adversely to certain antimicrobial agents. Those that should be avoided in the rabbit include lincomycin and clindamycin – the latter was used in this case. Other agents, such as procaine penicillin, are particularly contra-indicated in guinea pigs, rats and mice.

17 The bird's beak is deformed and overgrown. The appearance of the tail may indicate a feather problem, such as French moult. A deformed beak is sometimes a sequel to 'scaly face'.

18 No. While an excess of androgens leads to prostatic enlargement due to acinar hyperplasia, an excess of oestrogens can cause fibromuscular hyperplasia and squamous metaplasia of the duct system. Thus, prolonged oestrogen therapy for prostatic disease may **cause** prostatic enlargement rather than cure it. Similarly, Sertoli cell tumours of the testes may lead to prostatic enlargement.

19 (a) and (b) Isoflurane. With halothane, induction is little different but recovery is slower. Induction and recovery with methoxyflurane are slow.

(c) Methoxyflurane. This is an excellent analgesic, even at sub-anaesthetic levels. Isoflurane and halothane have only moderate analgesic properties.

(d) Isoflurane. However, all three volatile agents cause respiratory depression.

(e) Methoxyflurane. At clinically adequate doses blood pressure is well-maintained, but hypotension can still occur in the case of overdoses.

(f) Halothane. Halothane and isoflurane cause similar hypotension, but, while with isoflurane this is primarily due to peripheral vasodilation, halothane is more depressant to the myocardium.

20 (a) The clinical signs noted in this case are in themselves very suggestive of Cushing's disease. However, routine biochemistry and haematology are very useful as a preliminary to specific hormone testing in order to back up this supposition and to avoid overlooking any other disease condition which may be present.

(b) Considering the profile performed, the pointers which should be looked for with regard to Cushing's disease are as follows (in order of test listing rather than importance):

(i) **Low urea** due to anabolic (nitrogen-retaining) action of adrenocortical hormones.

(ii) **Raised glucose** due to excess glucocorticoids.

(iii) **Raised cholesterol.**

(iv) **Moderately high ALP** due to steroid-induced induction of a specific ALP isoenzyme (SIALP), produced in the liver.

(v) **Slight polycythaemia** (raised PCV), due to the effect of steroid hormones on erythropoietin production.

(vi) **'Steroid pattern' in WBCs** – this consists mainly of lymphopenia, eosinopenia and monocytosis. An absolute neutrophilia is occasionally seen, but usually any 'neutrophilia' is only relative, due to the lymphopenia.

(c) If strict attention was paid to the reference values quoted here, then only three of the relevant abnormalities could be claimed (cholesterol, ALP and monocytes).

(d) Although the first two (cholesterol and ALP) are quite important findings, they would hardly be sufficient to support the probability of Cushing's if all other pointers were completely absent. However, in this type of hormonal condition, test values can be highly significant **while still remaining within the 'normal' range**. If constituents are included where the results lie close to the reference limits in the appropriate direction, it can be seen that almost all the relevant features are demonstrated in this case (with the exception of the hyperglycaemia). This set of results in fact gives an extremely strong provisional diagnosis of Cushing's disease. In this condition no single result is pathognomonic – only a minority of cases demonstrate every abnormality, while **any** one, two or even three of these features, even the high ALP or the eosinopenia, may be absent in any given case. It is therefore important to cast the testing net as wide as possible to try to ascertain whether enough of the picture is present to justify this provisional diagnosis.

(e) Dynamic cortisol testing is essential to confirm the diagnosis. (Note that a single resting cortisol estimation is useless in this context.)

(f) The diagnosis can be considered to be provisional only until cortisol testing is undertaken; and drug treatment aimed at destroying adrenal tissue should not be contemplated without a reasonably certain diagnosis. Both the ACTH stimulation test and the low-dose (0.01 mg/kg) dexamethasone screening test are used for this purpose. The ACTH stimulation test is preferred because:

(i) It is unaffected by stress during the test, while the DXM test can become highly misleading if the patient is stressed.

(ii) It is quicker to perform.

(iii) Only two samples are required, as opposed to three, which makes it significantly cheaper.

(iv) Only the ACTH stimulation test is of any use in monitoring response to treatment, and if it is to be used for this purpose then a pre-treatment test is also necessary for comparison.

The high-dose (0.1 mg/kg) dexamethasone suppression test may be used after a diagnosis of Cushing's syndrome has been established with certainty using one of the other two tests, to distinguish between pituitary-dependent Cushing's and adrenal tumours. However, this is essential only in the event of an adrenal tumour being diagnosed and surgery contemplated; most cases are treated satisfactorily by medical means irrespective of the aetiology, and thus this step is often omitted.

An ACTH stimulation test was carried out in this patient and the results were Cortisol (pre-ACTH), 96 nmol/l (20–250); cortisol (2 h post-ACTH), 626 nmol/l.

In adrenal tumours the resting cortisol is usually moderately high with little further response to the ACTH, while pituitary-dependent cases usually start normal and show an exaggerated response to ACTH. Once the post-ACTH value exceeds 500 nmol/l, suspicions of Cushing's may be entertained, while values over 800–1000 nmol/l are virtually pathognomonic. In this case, while the post-ACTH value of 626 nmol/l did not reach this degree of absolute certainty, in conjunction with the very typical clinical signs and the highly suspicious routine biochemistry and haematology it was considered to be sufficiently diagnostic. Treatment with mitotane (o p' DDD) was instituted, with excellent results. Thirst declined to normal, nocturia ceased, the pendulous abdomen disappeared, and a normal hair coat began to re-grow.

21 (a) The dog is infected with *Filaroides osleri*, the canine lungworm. The parasite is not uncommon in dogs – such as greyhounds – kept in groups and is often subclinical. Where coughing is caused, it is invariably seen in dogs under 2 years of age.

(b) The diagnosis is best confirmed by bronchoscopy, where nodules may be seen at the tracheal bifurcation (*Figure 240*). The demonstration of larvae in the faeces is not always reliable and radiographs of the chest may not be diagnostic. Treatment with fenbendazole is effective, though may need to be extended beyond the normal 5-day course. In groups of dogs, other animals, especially the bitch and the litter mates, should also be treated.

22 (a) Subgingival calculus. It usually has a darker pigmentation than supragingival calculus and is more firmly attached to the cementum.

(b) It is the most destructive and irritant of the dental deposits, and must be removed during prophylaxis by scaling below the gingival margin in the pockets. If the pockets are too deep for proper débridement and post-operative care, extraction should be considered.

23 (a) Primary hereditary cataract.

(b) Labrador retriever.

(c) Do not breed from affected dogs or from their close relatives unless they have been examined and found free from the cataract at a reasonable age. Cataract in these breeds is due to a dominant gene but with considerable variation in age incidence.

24 (a) The 'finger test'.

(b) Underdevelopment. In a correctly developed film the background density should be so dark (black) that it is impossible to see a finger interposed between the film and the viewer. As a result of underdevelopment however, this film has a grey background and the finger is easily seen. The radiograph will have much reduced contrast as a result.

Underdevelopment is the most common fault seen with manual film processing and is due to the use of developer which is exhausted, diluted or too cold, or which is used for too short a time.

(c) Underdevelopment may be avoided by keeping the developer tank covered, by topping up with special replenisher solution, by frequent changes of developer, and by maintaining the developer at the correct temperature. Remember that developer will deteriorate with time even if it has not been used.

25 (a) A palisading periosteal reaction.

(b) Hypertrophic pulmonary osteopathy (Marie's disease).

(c) The condition is characterised by warm, painful, firm, non-oedematous, symmetrical swellings of all four feet and distal limbs. Animals are lame and reluctant to walk, The condition generally develops secondary to a thoracic mass (pulmonary tumours and granulomatous masses being the commonest causes), so there may be dyspnoea, cough or other signs referable to thoracic disease. Less commonly, the condition develops secondary to abdominal masses such as bladder tumours.

26 When you buy a bulldog you also buy the respiratory noises which go with it! Members of this breed are practically never quiet breathers and most show obstructive airway disease to a greater or lesser extent. The patient illustrated in *Figure 19* was a sensationally bad example and was afflicted by the following:

  (i) Stenotic nares (*Figure 241*).

  (ii) Soft palate hyperplasia.

  (iii) Eversion of the laryngeal ventricles (*Figure 242*).

  (iv) Inversion of the cuneiform appendages.

  (v) Glosso-epiglottic entrapment (*Figure 243*).

  (vi) Tracheal hypoplasia.

With the exception of (iv), all of the above were treated at the first surgical session. However, a bypass tracheotomy was needed during surgery and for 12 hours thereafter (*Figure 244*). The cuneiform inversion improved after resection to relieve the obstructions mentioned, but the tracheal hypoplasia proved to be a long-term, exercise-limiting factor. Tracheal hypoplasia is a condition exclusive to the English bulldog; it may be confirmed via a lateral radiograph of the neck and anterior thorax by comparing the width of the trachea with that of the cricoid or of the thoracic inlet (*Figure 245*).

27 (a) Pericardial effusion and cardiac tamponade are present (*Figure 20*).
(b) A mass, probably neoplastic, is visible, attached to the aorta (*Figure 21*).
The effusion is likely to be haemorrhage from the mass which, in this position, is probably an aortic body tumour. Congenital abnormalities of the mitral valve do occur occasionally in young Great Danes, but this is likely to be a case of dilated cardiomyopathy.

28 (a) *Microsporum canis*.
(b) Via systemic griseofulvin.
(c) Griseofulvin is strongly teratogenic, and should not be used if this stray cat might be pregnant.
(d) Clipping the cat's coat short and treating it topically with an antifungal wash.

29 The left ventricle is extremely dilated and thin-walled, as is the left atrium.

30 (a) A 'capped elbow' or acquired elbow bursa (hygroma).
(b) An acquired bursa occurs in response to repeated trauma and breakdown of the affected tissues. The inflammatory exudate eventually becomes enclosed in a well-delineated closed sac with a tough dense wall composed of granulation tissue and collagen. The inner layer of the sac is composed of flattened fibroblasts rather than true epithelium. Projections of tissue into the lumen of the cyst often give it a multilocular appearance.
(c) Infection and wound dehiscence. Continued trauma to the area must be prevented.

31 An oval soft-tissue dense mass the size of a melon is visible in the mid-ventral abdomen, displacing small intestines dorsally. This mass is well-defined and shows a small 'beak' cranioventrally. Cranial to the mass is food-filled pylorus. Both kidneys are visible dorsally. No normal splenic shadow is evident.
Diagnosis: splenic mass (due to the position of the mass and the 'beak' representing residual normal splenic tissue). The mass is most likely to be due to a haemangioma or haemangiosarcoma. Further diagnostic imaging tests would include chest radiography for metastases, and diagnostic ultrasound with fine-needle aspiration. This mass was a haemangiosarcoma.

32 (a) 'Feline neck lesions', 'feline resorption cavities'. The condition is usually extremely painful even though the animal may not exhibit obvious pain.
(b) By the time the cavities are diagnosed they may have destroyed a significant amount of tooth substance, and fracture of the crown can even result.
(c) To date, no restorative or palliative treatment affords a long-term or predictable prognosis of the affected teeth. Extractions are the treatment of choice.

33 (a) No – optic nerve hypoplasia is evident.
(b) A small grey optic disc with abnormal disc vessels. The condition was bilateral but the other eye was not severely affected and vision was present but defective.

34 (a) Anaesthetic death due to cardiac dysrhythmia, post-operative hypocalcaemic tetany, and recurrence of hyperthyroidism.
(b) Correct preparation of the patient for surgery is essential once the diagnosis has been confirmed by estimation of hormone levels. The cat should be rendered euthyroid by

medication with carbimazole (5 mg three times daily for 2 weeks). Should tachycardia persist after this therapy propranolol should be provided during the 2 days before surgery (2.5 mg twice daily).

Hypocalcaemia is the most frequent complication of this surgery and arises because of the intimate relationships of the parathyroid glands with the thyroids. Associated with each thyroid are two parathyroids. The cranial (external) lobe is usually obvious but the position of the internal parathyroid is very variable, ranging from the caudal pole to being buried within the thyroid tissue. Both lobes are obvious in *Figure 29*, but this is not often the case. Since the objective of surgery is to remove all of the thyroid tissue but to preserve the parathyroids with their vascular supply, many surgeons opt for an intra-capsular thyroidectomy technique, i.e., the thyroid tissue is teased away from the capsule, which is left *in situ* together with the parathyroids. However, this increases the risk of recurrence of hyperthyroidism.

The signs of hypocalcaemia include weakness, muscular tremors, twitching and convulsions; they are most likely to appear 24–72 hours after surgery. It is important **not** to provide calcium supplementation on the basis of laboratory data but to reserve this therapy for those cats which develop clinical signs. Sub-clinical hypocalcaemia is an important stimulus to parathyroid activity in the post-operative period.

35 (a) Malignant melanoma and squamous cell carcinoma.
(b) Examination of cytological material collected by fine needle or scraping is often diagnostic.
(c) Surgical resection of the affected digit.
(d) The prognosis is good for squamous cell carcinoma as distant metastasis is rare. It is guarded in malignant melanoma.

36 (a), (c) and (e). Aside from the well-known association of taurine deficiency and retinal lesions, it has recently been shown that many cases of cardiomyopathy in cats are responsive to taurine supplementation. Aortic thromboembolism is commonly associated with cardiomyopathy.

37 (a) Close inspection will probably reveal a perivulval dermatitis, especially in the skin folds dorsal and lateral to the vulva; the vulval lips may also be inflamed (*Figure 31*). Because of the painful nature of the condition, sedation or general anaesthesia may be necessary to attempt a thorough examination. The condition is sometimes claimed to be that of juvenile or hypoplastic vulva. In fact, in most cases the vulva **is** of a normal size, but – because the dorsal portion is covered by a fold of adjacent skin – casual examination may give the impression that it is abnormally small. Perivulval dermatitis has been said to occur most commonly in bitches which have been ovariectomised before puberty, but there is no evidence to support this; however, the condition occurs usually in bitches which are overweight.
(b) Provision of topical antibiotics and anti-inflammatory preparations may control the condition but many bitches resent their application and/or immediately lick them off. Surgical removal of the diseased tissue is usually necessary.

38 (a) This is probably an abscess of the dewlap. *Pasteurella multocida* is a prevalent organism in rabbits and can be associated with a range of infectious conditions.
(b) The abscess should be kept open, to facilitate drainage, and irrigated with an appropriate disinfectant or antimicrobial agent. The latter should be selected carefully on the basis of (i) sensitivity tests, and (ii) safety (some agents are toxic to rabbits).

Similar precautions should be taken if systemic agents are employed. Total excision of infected lesions is sometimes advisable.

39 (a) The most probable causes are hypothermia and/or too much anaesthetic (either the thiopentone, the methoxyflurane – or both). Some opioid drugs (particularly buprenorphine), if given at the end of anaesthesia, may delay recovery. Recovery from methoxyflurane is also slow. Cerebral oxygen deprivation as a result of airway obstruction, respiratory depression, failure of oxygen supply or circulatory failure will cause delayed return of consciousness, but this should have been detected during the monitoring of anaesthesia.

(b) The cat's temperature should be measured, and hypothermia corrected. Full anaesthetic monitoring should continue, and respiratory and cardiovascular support should be given if required. Warm fluid infusion will help to warm the cat and, by increasing renal flow, will also increase the elimination of many injected drugs, thus speeding recovery.

40 (a) A buffy coat smear is prepared to investigate abnormal white cells which may be present in such small numbers that they could be overlooked on a normal blood smear.

(b) Several mast cells, identifiable by the dark blue cytoplasmic granules and round nucleus, can be seen. Eosinophils are also evident, similar in appearance but with typical pink granules.

(c) The presence of mast cells in the blood is diagnostic of systemic mast cell tumours. It is possible that one or more of the skin nodules is a mast cell tumour, but whether the systemic tumours represent metastasis from one of these or have arisen separately within the reticulo-endothelial system is difficult to say.

(d) The prognosis is ultimately hopeless, as the systemic form of this disease is not usually responsive to treatment.

This bitch was put on a moderately high dose of prednisolone in an attempt to control the tumours. The vomiting improved somewhat but the polydipsia and weight loss continued. About 6 weeks after the initial diagnosis she became very depressed and refused all food, and the decision was taken to put her to sleep. At post-mortem examination, the spleen, liver and mesenteric lymph nodes were found to be packed with mast cells.

41 The lethargy may be the result of old age: female tarantulas can live for many years in captivity. A bare abdomen in spiders can be due to normal defensive behaviour: the insect rubs off 'hairs' (setae) with its legs and these can cause irritation to the skin or eyes of potential predators. In this case, however, the alopecia is more severe and is on the ventral, as well as the dorsal, surface of the abdomen. It is probably indicative of a physical injury or infection of the exoskeleton.

42 (a) This bitch is showing signs of urinary incontinence, with leakage of urine and secondary ulceration at the ventral commissure of the vulval lips.

(b) The conditions which may result in incontinence in this juvenile bitch are:

    (i) Ureteral ectopia (particularly in view of the breed).

    (ii) Congenital urethral sphincter mechanism incompetence.

    (iii) Intersexuality.

    (iv) Detrusor instability (e.g., bladder hypoplasia, urinary tract infection).

    (v) Neurogenic overflow incontinence (pervious urachus would result in incontinence through the umbilicus).

(c) Radiographic techniques should include intravenous urography and retrograde positive contrast vagino-urethrography. Urethrography alone would not detect an ectopic ureter terminating in the vagina, and pneumocystography is a waste of time in incontinence investigations, apart from its value in improving the contrast between distal ureters and bladder during intravenous urography.

43 (a) The condition is probably vaginal hyperplasia, frequently referred to as vaginal prolapse. The aetiology of the condition is unclear but it is suggested that it represents an abnormally intense response of vaginal tissue to oestrogenic stimulation during oestrus. The mass is not a true prolapse, but consists of oedematous and hyperplastic vaginal wall; it commonly arises only from the ventral vaginal wall, although it may involve the complete circumference of the vagina. The hyperplasia will regress at the end of oestrus.

(b) The tissue should be protected using creams and lubricants. Recurrence can be prevented by performing an ovariohysterectomy before the next oestrus. If the animal is required for breeding, the hyperplastic tissue must be removed during oestrus (there is no evidence that the condition is inherited).

44 (a) The IRT result was only very marginally abnormal, just into the equivocal range. EPI can be diagnosed with reasonable certainty only when the IRT is <2.5 ng/ml; animals with results in the range 2.5–4.9 ng/ml should be re-tested a few months later. Thus the original diagnosis of EPI was very suspect.

(b) The usual interpretation of a high bile acid result is either liver dysfunction or biliary obstruction. There is no specific association with hepatic carcinoma other than that this is one of the more common conditions associated with this finding in older patients (particularly in human patients – the origin of the misleading comment in this report was a medical laboratory technician in a 'veterinary' laboratory which had no veterinary surgeon on the staff). However, patients with portocaval shunts, acquired or congenital, also show very high plasma bile acid levels, and in a young dog a congenital shunt is by far the most likely reason for such a finding, particularly where there is a history of poor health. Closer inspection of the routine results tends to confirm this suspicion. While the abnormalities (slightly low albumin, slightly raised liver enzymes and marginally low urea) were not marked enough to lead to any firm conclusions by themselves, in conjunction with the bile acid result they take on an extra degree of significance.

(c) Initially, plasma ammonia (if feasible – patients usually have to travel to the laboratory for this test) and dynamic bile acids.

(d) Yes, these results confirm hyperammonaemia (the cause of the apparent CNS signs) and a portosystemic shunt.

(e) Bile acids are formed in the liver, excreted in the bile, reabsorbed from the small intestine and returned to the liver via the portal circulation. Thus high concentrations are not reached in the peripheral circulation under normal circumstances. However, in the presence of a portocaval shunt, blood from the portal vein empties directly into the posterior vena cava and enters the peripheral circulation. Thus after a meal, when bile acids are being reabsorbed, peripheral blood concentration of bile acids rise enormously.

(f) Portal angiography is necessary to visualise the abnormal vessel (patient ductus venosus), and an attempt to tie this off may be made immediately if the vessel is accessible.

(g) Prognosis is guarded. Possible complications include:

(i) Abnormal vessel entirely intra-hepatic and so inaccessible to surgery.

(ii) Insufficient portal circulation in the liver to take the diverted blood, either due to a primary abnormality which may have been the reason for the ductus venosus remaining patent in the first place, or which has developed as a result of delay in diagnosis/treatment. In this case severe intestinal congestion develops when attempts are made to tie off the abnormal vessel.

This dog could tolerate only a very small amount of constriction on the abnormal vessel. A temporary clinical improvement was gained after surgery, but about 3 months later the clinical signs returned with renewed severity and the dog was put to sleep.

45　(a) This is 'scaly face'.

(b) The causal organism, the mite *Cnemidocoptes*, can usually be demonstrated in a skin scraping or a biopsy.

46　All of them. Bladder catheterisation allows urine to exit from the body rather than enter the peritoneal cavity, and intravenous fluids have a 'flushing' effect in accelerating removal of toxins (urea, hydrogen and potassium ions) by the kidney. In these preliminary stages of treatment, fluids containing potassium are best avoided because of the risk of worsening the degree of hyperkalaemia. Intravenous bicarbonate is useful to correct the acidosis.

The most efficient method of correcting the metabolic consequences of bladder rupture is abdominal drainage (to remove the source of urea and hydrogen and potassium ions) and dialysis to reduce blood levels of the same toxins.

47　(a) A female ferret is called a 'jill' (a male is a 'hob').

(b) The significance of the vulval swelling is that ferrets are induced ovulaters and as a result, if not mated, can have a persistent oestrus. This in turn can lead to bone-marrow depression, anaemia and thrombocytopenia. Oestrus-associated bone-marrow depression is often fatal.

48　(a) The best 'monitor' of the anaesthetised animal is in fact the constant attention of an experienced anaesthetist (which can include an anaesthetic nurse). He/she should continually monitor the airway, breathing, circulation, and depth of anaesthesia.

(b) Respiratory rate, adequacy of airway and an indication of tidal volume can all be obtained by observation of the anaesthetic reservoir bag, and the colour of the mucous membranes indicates efficiency of ventilation. The circulation is best monitored by palpation of a peripheral pulse, monitoring of heart rate (the oesophageal stethoscope provides a simple but effective method), and observation of the colour of mucous membranes and of capillary refill time. The correct functioning of the anaesthetic machine and circuits (percentage of oxygen, adequacy of flow rates, efficacy of soda lime, circuit connections) also requires attention. The animal's temperature should be noted at intervals.

(c) The only limitation to the use of sophisticated monitors for all parameters is that of finance. Cardiovascular monitors (ECG, pulse monitors, arterial blood pressure monitoring) should have priority, as respiration is more easily assessed by observation. Pulse oximetry, by measuring the saturation of haemoglobin in the peripheral tissues, gives an indication of both respiratory and circulatory efficiency.

49 (a) Bilateral medial patellar luxation.

(b) The possible causes include coxa valga; lateral bowing of the distal femur; medial bowing of the proximal tibia; medial rotation of the tibial crest; hypoplasia of the medial trochlear ridge; and aplasia of the trochlea.

(c) The condition usually occurs in the toy breeds such as the Yorkshire Terrier, Chihuahua, Miniature and Toy poodle, Pekingese, Pomeranian and Cavalier King Charles spaniel. Occasionally, it is found in larger breeds such as Chow Chows and Labrador retrievers.

50 (a) The fluid should undergo:

(i) **Cytological analysis.** This will demonstrate an acute inflammatory response usually without any micro-organisms.

(ii) **Biochemical analysis.** This will demonstrate an elevated bilirubin level. Other tests should include urea and creatinine levels to check for the presence of a bladder rupture.

(b) The appearance of the fluid is consistent with a bile peritonitis, and the fluid's most likely cause is **extrahepatic biliary trauma** (rupture of the gall bladder or, more likely, rupture of the common bile duct).

(c) A variety of surgical procedures may be indicated, including:

(i) **Cholecystectomy** in the case of gall bladder rupture.

(ii) **Repair of the common bile duct** in the case of damage to the duct by debriding the two ends of the duct and anastomosing them over a stent using fine (4/0–6/0) absorbable suture material.

(iii) **Cholecystoenterostomy** may be performed where repair of the duct is not feasible. The gall bladder is mobilised and anastomosed in a two-layer repair to the small intestine (duodenum, jejunum).

(d) Complications of biliary surgery include:

(i) **Stenosis of the bile duct** leading to icterus.

(ii) **Leakage** at the repair site leading to ongoing biliary peritonitis.

(iii) Cholecystoenterostomy may be complicated by **stenosis of the stoma site** leading to icterus.

51 (a) A 'knocked-up' toe. It is a subluxation of the distal interphalangeal joint.

(b) It is due usually to rupture of the deep digital flexor tendon. Occasionally, it occurs as a result of an avulsion fracture of the tuberosity of the third phalanx at the insertion of this tendon. In both instances, the dorsal elastic ligament of the third phalanx pulls the toe proximally, since the opposing pull of the deep digital flexor tendon is lost.

(c) A 'dropped toe' is due to a rupture of the superficial digital flexor tendon. This tendon inserts on the second rather than the third phalanx.

52 (a) Trauma to the tooth has severed its blood supply, causing necrosis of the pulp.

(b) Teeth with such an injury may have a pink or violet tip, or the whole tooth may exibit a grey hue.

(c) Even though no exposure of the pulp has taken place, periapical pathology may result. Root canal treatment can offer a predictable and preventative treatment.

53 (a) Regular sinus arrest is present and is probably an exaggeration of sinus arrhythmia. The pauses are greater than twice the R–R intervals. The rate is slow (40 beats/minute).

(b) This bradycardia could well be associated with CNS disease and increased intra-cranial pressure.

54 (a) There is blurring of the trabecular pattern and mottled patchy densities in the medullary cavity. The endosteal margins are less distinct. These changes are typical of panosteitis or enostosis.
(b) Haematological and biochemical parameters are usually within normal limits. Neutrophilia, monocytosis and lymphopaenia have been recorded, probably reflecting stress.
(c) This condition is seen in many of the large breed dogs but occurs especially in male German shepherd dogs.

55 (a) Vesico-ureteral reflux and iatrogenic bladder rupture have occurred, although the spillage of contrast medium around the bladder neck makes it difficult to rule out reflux of contrast medium from the prostatic urethra into ectopic ureters.
(b) The investigator was ignorant of the presence of marked bladder hypoplasia, and bladder capacity was exceeded during the retrograde contrast study.

56 (a) Perianal fistulae (anal furunculosis).
(b) Surgical débridement of fistulae together with the removal of any underlying systemic disease.
(c) At best the prognosis is guarded, lesions often recurring.

57 (a) Malocclusions – overgrowth of cheek teeth, forming a bridge which traps the tongue and causes dysphagia.
(b) Infectious agents are probably not involved. Various nutritional deficiencies have been implicated, including a paucity of hay or other fibre which the animal can chew. Broken teeth and jaw abnormalities can also be responsible. Genetic factors are probably involved in some cases.

58 Unwanted pregnancies are best terminated by ovariohysterectomy 2–3 weeks after the end of oestrus. Alternatively, oral or parentral oestrogen therapy may be given to bitches which may be required for subsequent breeding. Such therapy is effective only when administered up to 5 days after mating, and may induce bone marrow suppression and predispose to pyometra; bitches may also continue to show signs of oestrus after oestrogen administration.
Canine corpora lutea are relatively unresponsive to prostaglandin administration for the first 2–3 weeks of pregnancy. After this, repeated administration of low doses or single administration of high doses of prostaglandin can be used to terminate pregnancy. The adverse effects of such drugs (vomiting, diarrhoea, hypothermia) means that they are not commonly used for this purpose. Corticosteroids, too, will effect abortion, but the high doses and the necessity for repeated administration make this method both impractical and inadvisable.

59 A primary malignant bone tumour, most likely to be an osteosarcoma. This example is very osteoproductive.

60 (a) Tarsal valgus of the right hindlimb.
(b) Premature closure of the lateral aspect of the distal tibial growth plate.
(c) The type of treatment depends upon the age of the dog. If it is under 6 months of age and the distal tibial growth plate is still active, it is possible to correct the deformity by slowing growth on the medial aspect of the limb using a transepiphyseal bridging technique. Alternatively, the activity of the lateral aspect of the growth plate can be encouraged by hemi-circumferential periosteal transection. In the skeletally mature dog, the deformity is corrected by an osteotomy of the distal tibia.

61 (a) The ECG is normal.
(b) Examine the abdomen carefully – German shepherds are particularly prone to splenic haemangiosarcoma, which results in recurrent abdominal haemorrhage. However, remember that one normal ECG does not rule out cardiac disease or intermittent arrhythmias.

62 (a) The lower canine has suffered a longitudinal fracture. The crack extends through the root as well as the crown. Purulent exudate from the infected root canal is seen discharging through the fracture line.
(b) The tooth is unsavable. Extraction is mandatory.

63 (a) The cat has anterior mediastinal (thymic) lymphosarcoma with compression of the oesophagus at the thoracic inlet and the accumulation of pleural fluid.
(b) Radiography confirms the presence of an anterior mediastinal mass and fluid. Thoracentesis reveals typically a non-viscous translucent bloodstained fluid containing large numbers of lymphocytes and lymphoblasts. Occasionally, the fluid is chylous. The majority of cases of this form of lymphosarcoma are feline leukaemia virus (FeLV) positive. In some cases the presence of an anterior mediastinal mass can be appreciated by the loss of 'spring' on compression of the anterior thorax.

64 The snake is about to shed (slough) its skin: an opacity of the 'spectacles' (scales covering the eyes) is a sign that shedding is imminent. The owner should also be advised that **sand snakes are** rear-fanged and therefore **venomous**. They do not require a licence in Britain but care should be taken when handling them.

65 (a) The only real abnormality here is the regenerative anaemia, and it seems probable that anaemia was the reason for the collapse. However, a PCV of 0.32 is not nearly low enough to cause collapse, and indeed the dog was bright and alert at the time the blood sample was collected. It is therefore probable that the PCV was considerably lower at the time of the collapse.
(b) Given the regenerative RBC picture, the anaemia must be either haemolytic or haemorrhagic. There are no obvious signs of haemorrhage in the results – no hypochromasia, no thrombocytosis, and albumin is not particularly low – but neither are there any real indications of haemolysis. There was no haemolysis or icterus evident in the blood sample, and no distorted RBCs. In addition, it is highly unlikely that a dog would spontaneously recover from a severe acute haemolytic crisis to virtual clinical normality and a PCV of over 0.30 – twice! On the other hand, an acute haemorrhagic

episode where the bleeding occurs into a body cavity (usually the abdomen), so that the blood is not lost from the body but can be reabsorbed, may be followed by just such a rapid recovery, and this sort of episode does tend to recur. This also explains the lack of hypoalbuminaemia or hypochromasia, as each is caused by actual loss of blood constituents (protein and iron) from the body.

(c) The lesion usually responsible for intermittent intra-abdominal haemorrhage is the haemangiosarcoma. This is quite common in older German shepherd dogs, and the majority occur in the spleen. The liver is the second most common site, but the normal liver enzymes in this case suggest that the liver is not involved at this stage.

(d) The above hypothesis may be confirmed by the demonstration of free blood in the abdomen by paracentesis. However, exploratory laparotomy will be necessary to establish exactly the site and nature of the lesion.

(e) Short-term prognosis depends on the site of the haemangiosarcoma. If it is splenic, splenectomy will produce an excellent clinical improvement in the short term; however, tumours involving other organs such as the liver can be more difficult to deal with surgically. In any case, the medium to long term prognosis is extremely poor as these tumours virtually always recur, often because the problem lesion was itself a secondary tumour from a small primary elsewhere in the body, and it is only a matter of time before further secondaries appear.

Paracentesis in this case produced a fluid indistinguishable from blood (PCV 0.40) from two different sites on the abdomen. Exploratory laparotomy revealed traces of free blood in the abdominal cavity, and a typical haemangiosarcoma which appeared to have undergone recent rupture was present on the spleen. No other lesions were seen on any other organs. A splenectomy was performed and post-operative recovery was uneventful. The dog remained well for about 5 months, but then another episode of pallor and collapse occurred. About 2 weeks after this he was found dead in his basket one morning. At post-mortem examination the abdomen was full of clotted blood, and the remains of a ruptured haemangiosarcoma were evident on one of the liver lobes.

66 (a) The condition is pilonidal sinus, an embryological mishap in which foci of dermal tissue are drawn into the deeper layers of the neck when the neurectoderm of the neural plate migrates from the surface to form the spinal cord. Suppuration develops from the buried dermal elements which can lie at any level from the subcutis to the meninges.

(b) Knowledgeable breeders check newborn puppies for the tell-tale tufting of the hair and for the palpable cords of the sinus tracts which are usually multiple. Treatment necessitates the complete excision of the buried dermal tissues. Pre-surgical radiography using contrast medium to outline the extent of the sinus tracts is advisable. An example of an excised specimen is illustrated in *Figure 246*.

(c) Rhodesian Ridgeback (in which the condition arises almost exclusively).

67 Individual animals have different requirements but expected halothane concentrations would be in the region of (a) 1–2%, (b) 0.65–1%, and (c) 1.3–2%.

As the dog is on a non-rebreathing circuit the concentration of halothane delivered is that set at the vaporiser. The Minimal Alveolar Concentration (MAC) of halothane (that is, the alveolar concentration necessary to prevent movement in response to a painful stimulus in 50% of animals) in the dog has been measured as from 0.87–1%. Usually, 1.5 MAC is necessary to maintain anaesthesia, but up to 2 MAC may be required in some individuals to prevent response to painful surgery. Thus, in (a), 1.5–2

MAC may be necessary. Other anaesthetic and sedative drugs reduce the MAC of halothane by variable amounts. Acepromazine reduces MAC by up to 50%, and lasts the duration of the anaesthetic. Thiopentone further reduces the concentration of halothane required, thus the reduced requirement in (b). However, the action of propofol is so short that, 10–20 minutes after its administration, it has little influence on the concentration of halothane required for maintenance (c).

68 (a) Sarcoptic mange.
(b) Multiple scrapings taken from likely sites (non-traumatised papulocrustous lesions on pinnae, elbows, hocks and Achilles tendon area) reveal mites in 50–80% of untreated cases.
(c) If infestation with *Sarcoptes scabiei* mites is indicated by the history and examination, then six weekly dips in gamma-benzene hexachloride will allow this condition to be ruled out.

69 (a) A malleolar shearing injury of the medial hock joint.
(b) The medial malleolus of the tibia; the medial aspects of the talus, the central and second tarsal bones and the second metetarsal bone; the long and short medial collateral ligaments and the overlying soft tissues.
(c) Joint culture. Thorough débridement and joint lavage. Radiography to demonstrate the full extent of the bony damage. The collateral ligaments are replaced using three bone screws and two figure-of-eight braided polyester sutures. One screw is placed in the distal tibia at the origin of the collateral ligaments and, the remaining two are placed in the talus at the insertions of the long and short collateral ligaments, respectively. The repair is protected with a transarticular external fixator for approximately a month, during which time the wound is dressed daily and encouraged to heal by second intention.

70 (i) The tube head window must be fitted with an aluminium filter to remove low-energy X-rays which are a potential hazard to the patient and radiographer. The thickness of the filter will depend on the maximum kV of the machine, but for most machines in veterinary use it will be 2.0 mm A1. Some older machines may have had the filter removed, but this can be checked by an X-ray engineer.
(ii) The machine must have a light to show when it is 'in a state of readiness to produce X-rays' and a second light which illuminates during exposure.
(iii) The exposure button must be on a cable which is at least 2 m long, and must be of a type such that release of the button in an emergency automatically terminates the exposure.
(iv) Some means of collimation must be attached to the tube head, allowing the X-ray beam to be confined to within the borders of the film. A light beam diaphragm is strongly recommended and is a legal requirement if patients are ever held for radiography.

In addition, the machine must be serviced annually and the service records kept for possible inspection by Health and Safety Executive Inspectors.

71 (a) 'Sore hocks' (pododermatitis), due probably to a combination of hard surfaces and a rabbit that is overweight.
(b) Secondary infection may have occured.

(c) Treatment is a combination of (i) topical treatment by débridement, cleaning and (possibly) bandaging; (ii) provision of a softer substrate; and (iii), reducing the animal's weight.

72   (a) Giardiasis is the most probable diagnosis in this case.
(b) Confirmation of diagnosis is difficult, as the organism is not shed at all times, so multiple samples may be necessary. Fresh faecal smears are required to detect trophozoites, but the oocysts may be detected following zinc sulphate flotation. Asymptomatic carriers do occur, so it may be wise to treat all cats in the house.
(c) Oocysts can persist in the environment, so disinfection may be required to prevent reinfection of newly introduced cats.

73   (a) This is a case of Addison's disease. In the dog, it is caused usually by an auto-immune destruction of the adrenal cortex, and the peak age of onset for auto-immune conditions is 3–6 years.
(b) An ACTH stimulation test is the appropriate confirmation of this diagnosis. Cortisol level in Addison's cases is <100 nmol/l with little or no increase (often a decrease) post-ACTH. Frequently, no cortisol is detectable in either sample.
(c) Isotonic saline i/v in large quantities. This will correct the hypovolaemia (which will improve the renal function), reduce the hyperkalaemia by dilution and, as a result of the improved renal function, improve the hyponatraemia. Dexamethasone (at least 2 mg/kg) should be added to the infusion, but not until the second sample of the ACTH test has been collected. Dextrose saline, too, is effective in most cases of Addison's disease, and may be even more effective than isotonic saline in lowering the potassium – but, since a proportion of cases are severely hyponatraemic, this is best avoided as it will worsen hyponatraemia. Solutions containing potassium are contra-indicated for obvious reasons.
(d) The initial biochemistry showed evidence of a degree of pre-renal renal dysfunction (raised urea with normal or disproportionately low creatinine) which was probably of circulatory origin. This phenomenon is caused by either very severe dehydration or poor cardiac output – in Addison's disease both factors are involved. The raised plasma proteins pointed to dehydration and this combination of circumstances might have suggested Addison's disease. Where there is evidence of a pre-renal renal insufficiency with no other obvious cause (e.g. severe congestive heart disease), especially in younger dogs, sodium and potassium should always be measured as a precaution.
(e) Addison's disease is characterised by an extraordinarily severe hypovolaemia as a consequence of renal sodium wasting caused by lack of aldosterone. This hypovolaemia leads to extremely poor peripheral capillary perfusion, which in turn leads to peripheral hypothermia and in particular to cold extremities. This disturbs thermoregulation, trapping metabolic heat deep in the body, and is the probable reason for the core hyperthermia noted in this case.
This dog made a dramatic clinical improvement on the treatment outlined above. An ACTH stimulation test performed before starting steroid therapy revealed no detectable cortisol in either sample. He was discharged on 0.2 mg fludrocortisone acetate and 6 mg prednisolone per day orally, plus 2 g additional salt added to his food. Three weeks after discharge plasma sodium was 144 mmol/l and potassium 4.9 mmol/l. The dog remains well.

74   (a) The cat shows evidence of concurrent Horner's syndrome and facial palsy. The signs present are all on the cat's right side (left in *Figure 60*) and comprise enophthal-

mos, ptosis, protrusion of the third eyelid, narrowing of the palpebral fissure, relative pupillary constriction, and drooling from the corner of the mouth.

(b) Although Horner's syndrome can arise through lesions interfering with the function of the sympathetic pathways at any level from the brainstem via the cervical spinal cord, the rostral thoracic nerve roots, cervical sympathetic trunk, middle ear to the retro-bulbar area, the only site at which both the facial nerve and the sympathetic fibres are at all adjacent is the middle ear. Even so, the facial nerve is relatively protected by bone until it emerges from the stylomastoid foramen which opens immediately caudal to the middle ear. The post-ganglionic sympathetic fibres are vulnerable to insult within the middle ear, where they run over the promontory protected only by a layer of periosteum. Thus, the most likely explanation for the cat's condition is an aggressive middle ear tumour or surgically induced nerve damage. A careful otoscopic examination of the pretympanic section of the ear canal combined with radiographs of the petrous temporal bone would be helpful in arriving at a definitive diagnosis.

The cat in *Figure 60* had recently been subjected to a total ear canal ablation and lateral bulla osteotomy for the removal of middle ear polyps. The Horner's syndrome pre-existed the surgery through compression of the sympathetic nerve fibres by the polyps, and the facial palsy resulted from stretching of the nerve trunk during the operation. Both deficits resolved within 3 months of surgery.

(c) Cats with middle ear disease are more prone to Horner's syndrome than dogs because the sympathetic fibres in the latter species are less superficial, and expansive lesions in the middle ear are not common. The facial nerve of the cat is more likely to be stretched during retraction for lateral bulla osteotomy simply because of the size of the head.

75 (a) The incorrect incisor relationship seen in *Figure 61* is due to the lower arch being crowded. This has resulted in some of the lower incisors being pushed labially and the upper incisors being trapped lingually.

(b) No treatment should be considered for this genetically related abnormality.

76 The stereotyped behaviour was due probably to a dull and unenriched environment. Old-fashioned featureless cages are not suitable for parrots, which are gregarious and active birds.

The poor plumage may have been attributable to a nutritionally inadequate diet. Parrots housed in old-fashioned cages are often still fed on a basic diet of sunflower seeds, which are deficient in lysine and vitamin A, and have a suboptimum calcium: phosphorus ratio.

77 (a) No. Post-inflammatory retinopathy.

(b) Chorioretinitis with hyper-reflectivity and pigmentation in the centre. Note asymmetry of the lesion and only one eye was affected. No visual defect.

78 (a) The bitch's vagina is very long (up to 30 cm). In the majority of bitches it is therefore not possible to palpate the cervix *per vaginam* or inspect the cervix using conventional auriscopes. Paediatric proctoscopes or fiberoptic endoscopes are necessary for canine vaginoscopy. The caudal end of the dorsal median fold of vaginal mucosa, which runs backwards from the cervix, is often mistakenly identified as the cervix. The vaginal and cervical mucosa change during the oestrous cycle.

(b) The progressive changes of mucosal oedema and mucosal shrinkage allow the identification of the bitch's fertile period. The procedure may also be useful for examinations during parturition, and for investigations of vaginal strictures and abnormal discharges.

79 (a) The important clinical signs are bowing of the legs and soiling of the cloacal region. The bird has osteodystrophy (metabolic bone disease) due to a low calcium: high phosphorus intake.
(b) The condition could have been prevented by not feeding an all-meat diet, which is low in calcium.

80 (a) *Figure 66* has been recorded at the level of the chordae tendinae and *Figure 67* at the level of the mitral valve.
(b) Most authors agree that the normal canine range for fractional shortening is 25–40%, recorded at the level of the chordae tendinae.
(c) The formula is:

$$\frac{\text{Diastolic diameter} - \text{systolic diameter}}{\text{Diastolic diameter}} \times 100$$

81 (a) Legg Calve Perthes disease (avascular necrosis of the femoral head).
(b) The major vascular supply to the femoral head is via the capsular vessels. These originate from the cranial and caudal circumflex femoral arteries and from the cranial and caudal gluteal vessels.
(c) Possible surgical approaches to the hip joint include the cranio-lateral, the dorsal (either with osteotomy of the greater trochanter or transection of the gluteal muscles), the caudal and the ventral. The cranio-lateral approach is most suitable for femoral head and neck excision.

82 (a) This bitch is hypothyroid, a condition which is associated with lymphocytic thyroiditis.
(b) Diagnosis of hypothyroidism is suspected on the clinical signs and an elevated blood cholesterol level and confirmed by the demonstration of low blood T4 levels. The underlying pathology can be demonstrated only following biopsy and histopathology. Lymphocytic thyroiditis is an immune-mediated disease which typically affects young females. As such, it differs from 'classic' hypothyroidism, presumed to be associated with thyroid atrophy, and recognised in middle-aged or older animals showing bilateral alopecia with lethargy. However, treatment is similar and is based on thyroid replacement therapy.

83 (a) Haemorrhage is still occurring from one or more placental sites which have not completely involuted (so-called sub-involution). The cause of the condition is unknown. Neither ecbolic agents nor antibiotics are an effective treatment.
(b) Haemorrhage may persist until the next oestrus, after which it will resolve. Blood loss is rarely severe enough to necessitate ovariohysterectomy or transfusions.

84 There are two possible diagnoses:
(a) Subcutaneous emphysema, due to traumatic damage to an internal air sac.
(b) Grossly distended cervico-cephalic air sacs. The sacs, which lie at the back of the skull, are usually very small and not visible. The cause of distension is unclear but it may be a sequel to respiratory disease.

85   (a) An RPA is a Radiation Protection Advisor.

(b) The RPA is someone outside the practice who is appointed to advise on the way in which the practice should operate its radiography set-up in order to comply with the Ionising Radiations Regulations 1985. Most RPAs are either holders of the Diploma in Veterinary Radiology or hospital physicists. All practices must appoint an RPA unless they can show that they fulfill each of five criteria laid down in the Regulations.

The RPA will define the extent of the 'controlled area' and advise on warning signs and notices, often taking measurements during trial exposures to ensure that excessive levels of radiation are not detected in adjacent rooms. He or she will draw up the Local Rules (including the System of Work) for the practice which will describe the procedures for radiography to ensure the safety of all concerned. These include artificial restraint of patients for radiography and the circumstances in which they may be held; the personnel allowed to work with radiation; the use of protective clothing; dosimetry; the maintenance of equipment; and the keeping of radiography records.

86   (a) The lesions are dry gangrene, the result of frost-bite.

(b) Birds in aviaries are prone to this condition, especially if there is no heating during the winter or the perches are made of metal. Prevailing winds may render part of an otherwise well insulated aviary very cold.

87   (a) The history and clinical signs are consistent with **cowpox infection**, the multiple lesion being secondary to an initial skin infection some 2 weeks before.

(b) Confirmation of the diagnosis is by virus isolation or electronmicroscopy of scab material. Serology may be used in recovered animals. Systemic disease is uncommon but may follow treatment with corticosteroids, or immunosuppression, e.g. FIV infection.

(c) Treatment with antibiotics may be needed to control secondary bacterial infection but lesions usually heal without therapy. The infection is zoonotic and while human infection from cats is uncommon, occuring usually through skin abrasions, appropriate care should nevertheless be taken and the owners warned.

88   (a) Tranquillisers are drugs which relieve nervousness without making the animal sleepy. Sedatives make the animal sleepy, but it is still easily aroused, while hypnotics induce sleep.

(b) With some drugs the categories may merge, higher doses increasing effects, but others are more specific. An understanding of the categories enables the veterinary surgeon to recognise the limitations of the drugs used. Thus, acepromazine (a tranquilliser) is often very effective in nervous animals, but ineffective (at any dose) in the vicious dog.

89   (a) Conditions which produce an inability to **close** the mouth are few but include temporomandibular joint (TMJ) luxation, fracture of the horizontal and vertical mandibular rami, and mandibular neurapraxia. The cause here is thought to be damage to the mandibular branch of the trigeminal nerve by overstretching of the mouth or excessive load-carrying. (The patient was a frustrated footballer!)

(b) The alignment of the jaws appears to be symmetrical, and bilateral TMJ luxation is very rare. Unilateral TMJ luxation produces an obvious deviation of the mandible **away** from the side of dislocation. Mandibular fracture will be suspected if there is blood in the mouth or resentment when the mandible is manipulated; dogs which have sustained this trauma are usually not keen to eat. In mandibular neurapraxia the alignment of the jaws is symmetrical and the mouth can be closed passively without distress to the patient.

(c) Conservative treatment is effective and includes supporting the jaws in a closed position with a muzzle and hand-feeding from a height. Resolution can be expected within 7–10 days.

90 (a) The femoral head and acetabulum have been replaced by Richard's Canine II Hip Prostheses.

(b) Any disabling hip disease, i.e. dogs with lameness, exercise intolerance, altered locomotor function or pain attributable to the hip joint are all candidates for a total hip replacement. They should be skeletally mature, free from systemic disease or infection, and should not have other orthopaedic or neurological problems.

(c) Dislocation of the prostheses; infection; loose acebabular and/or femoral components due to bone-cement or cement-prosthesis interface failure; fractures and sciatic neuropraxia. In one large series the overall complication rate was 6.3%.

91 (a) In cases where a bleeding disorder is evident, full haematology is essential. Platelet counts cannot be done on postal samples; however, a visual assessment of platelet numbers on the blood film can be quite adequate for diagnosis and should always be a routine part of a complete haematological examination. Prothrombin time and activated partial thromboplastin time, however, do give acceptable results on postal samples.

(b) Tests which can be done only in the physical presence of the patient include:

  (i) Clotting time (tests for the integrity of the 'cascade' process).

  (ii) Clot retraction (tests platelet function, mainly).

  (iii) Bleeding time (also tests platelet function, but is perhaps best avoided unless absolutely necessary, as a 1-cm cut on the inside of the pinna is not particularly desirable in a patient with a severe bleeding problem).

(c) In this case, the postal results proved quite adequate for diagnosis, as the visual assessment of the blood smear provided clear evidence of thrombocytopenia.

(d) All other bone marrow cell lines are quite normal and the RBC picture is regenerative, so this is not a case of bone marrow aplasia. Given the age and sex of the patient, the sudden onset of the condition and the absence of any other signs of severe illness (which might raise the question of disseminated intravascular coagulation), the overwhelming probability is auto-immune thrombocytopenia. This could be confirmed if necessary by testing the serum for anti-platelet antibody.

(e) Treatment is by immunosuppressive doses of prednisolone, as for AIHA, routinely 1 mg/kg b.i.d. until clinical improvement is seen, and then withdrawing gradually over 3–4 weeks. The majority of cases of auto-immune thrombocytopenia respond very well and an increase in platelet numbers is usually appreciable in less than a week.

No test for anti-platelet antibody was done in this patient as the diagnosis was considered to be reasonably certain. By 1 week after the start of treatment the petechiation had virtually disappeared and the owner reported no sign of blood in the urine. Platelets were graded as 'adequate' on the blood film. Prednisolone was gradually withdrawn as described above and the bitch remained well for 8 months, at which time a repeat of the petechiation occurred. This was again successfully treated as described.

92 Possibilities include a feather cyst (*Hypopteronosis cystica*), an abscess, a haematoma, and a neoplasm. The diagnosis of a feather cyst is confirmed when the lesion is bisected (*Figure 247*), exposing a mass of keratin. Feather cysts occur because feathers fail to erupt properly through the skin. The condition may be inherited.

93 (a) Comedones containing abnormal deposits of melanin pigment.

(b) Colour mutant alopecia.

(c) Yes. This condition is a likely sequel to the dilute coat colour, and is therefore considered hereditary.

94 (a) This cat has extraperitoneal, or dry, feline infectious peritonitis (FIP).

(b) The age and presenting signs are typical; the latter are associated with a meningo-encephalitis and in this case an iritis. The diagnosis may be supported by serology, where a high coronavirus titre is consistent with FIP. However, serology is not always helpful, with interpretation of moderate titres particularly difficult. The demonstration of virus itself is not at present available for diagnosis. Diagnosis is usually confirmed at post-mortem examination, although in some cases involvement of other organs, such as kidneys or liver, may offer the opportunity for biopsy. The differential diagnosis includes spongiform encephalopathy, although present evidence suggests that this occurs typically in older cats, as do neoplasms of the CNS. Cases of ischaemic or infectious encephalopathies due to other agents are reported but rare. Thiamin (vitamin B1) deficiency is also uncommon.

95 (a) No. Multifocal retinal dysplasia.

(b) Grey branching retinal folds in the tapetal fundus superior to the optic disc. No visual defect.

96 While the apparent obstruction may be due to urolithiasis, it may result alternatively from a tortuous groove of the caudal os penis (which may prevent passage of a catheter, but not urine), a urethral stricture (usually following previous urethrotomies) or, rarely, a urethral foreign body or a tumour of the caudal os penis.

97 (a) The common name for enamel hypoplasia or amelogenesis imperfecta (which is the condition depicted in *Figure* 79) is 'distemper teeth'. It is caused not by distemper, however, but by inherited factors, or through systemic disturbance like a general infection, pyrexia, etc. during the period of enamel formation of the teeth in question.

(b) Usually the condition has no significance other than aesthetical.

(c) Any restorative treatment may be more traumatic than the condition itself and usually is only temporary in its prognosis.

98 (a) There is destruction of the intervertebral disc and the adjacent vertebral end plates. New bone formation on the ventral aspect of the vertebrae is evident. This is typical of a bacterial infection causing a discospondylitis.

(b) The major sign is back pain. Lameness is usually evident; less frequently, there may be neurological signs such as ataxia, paralysis and urinary incontinence.

(c) Pulmonary arterial thrombi and glomerulonephritis have been reported as complications.

99 (a) Squamous cell carcinoma (SCC) arises in elderly cats at sites which are poorly protected from the carcinogenic effects of ultra-violet radiation in sunlight. Thus, the ear tips, eyelid margins and rhinarium are vulnerable, especially when these areas are coloured white, i.e. when there is no pigmental protection either. At the rhinarium, SCC is as often erosive as proliferative, but the diagnosis should be confirmed by biopsy.

(b) The treatment options available include radiotherapy, resection of the nasal planum, and cryosurgery. Cryotherapy offers a practicable modality, although recurrence is possible with all three techniques. The tumour should be subjected to three freeze/thaw cycles using a closed probe cooled by liquid nitrogen or liquid nitrous oxide. The extent of the cryolesion is checked using hypodermic thermocouples (*Figure 248*). A good cosmetic effect can be achieved (*Figure 249*), although the successful treatment of long-standing and extensive lesions may necessitate a larger ice-ball and the loss of a wider area of tissue by cryonecrosis.

100   The technique of choice is the **double-contrast cystogram**, in which a small amount of a positive-contrast agent is used to demonstrate the mucosal surface, and then the bladder is distended with negative contrast (usually air) in order to show wall thickness and filling defects. The positive-contrast agent should be a low-concentration water-soluble iodine medium such as diatrizoate (Urografin 150; Schering).

Under sedation or general anaesthesia, the bladder is catheterised and completely drained of urine. A small amount (2–10 ml depending on patient size) of the positive-contrast medium is instilled. The bladder is then filled with air using a syringe and three-way tap until it is gently turgid. Lateral and ventrodorsal radiographs should be taken, ensuring that the hindlimbs are drawn well back for the lateral view. After the procedure the bladder is emptied of air and positive contrast.

101   Yes. Urease-producing organisms (e.g. staphylococci, *Proteus*) result in increased urinary concentrations of ammonium ions, one of the constituents of triple phosphate and struvite calculi. In addition, the increase in ammonium ion concentration results in a more alkaline urine, in which these types of calculi are less soluble.

102   (a) Sertoli cell tumour.
(b) Lack of libido and attractiveness to male dogs.
(c) Oestrogen-related bone-marrow suppression with anaemia.
(d) Surgical removal of **both** testicles. (There is an increased incidence of Sertoli cell tumour in contra-lateral testicles of affected dogs.)

103   (a) Both, the high percentage of conjugated bilirubin and the more striking elevation of serum alkaline phosphatase when compared to analine transferase are consistent with a post-hepatic jaundice. Liver function, as crudely assessed by urea and albumin levels, is adequate and there is no evidence of a pre-hepatic, or haemolytic, jaundice.
(b) In a dog of this age the most likely cause of obstruction is neoplasia, either a pancreatic carcinoma or a bile-duct cholangiosarcoma. Chronic pancreatitis is an uncommon cause of obstruction and bile duct calculi are rare.

104   (a) This dog has an **oesophageal foreign body** (chop bone) lodged immediately cranial to the cardia.
(b) This instrument is an open illuminated **oesophagoscope**/bronchoscope.
(c) It can be used to visualise the foreign body, whose **retrieval** can then be effected by means of crocodile forceps passed through the scope.
(d) Oesophageal foreign bodies have a number of possible **complications**, including:
   (i) **Oesophagitis**
   (ii) **Oesophageal perforation** causing pneumomediastinum, mediastinitis, pleural effusion and aortic rupture.
   (iii) **Oesophageal stricture** (*Figure 85*).

105 (a) Acepromazine is a phenothiazine drug which is primarily a tranquilliser, although it does have some limited sedative properties. Xylazine and medetomidine are sedative/hypnotics.

(b) Acepromazine causes vasodilation which results in hypotension. Most animals given acepromazine have normal or slightly raised heart rates, but a few individual dogs, especially those of the boxer breed, may have severe bradycardia and may collapse. The drug has minimal respiratory effects, has anti-emetic actions amd mild anti-histamine properties. When used as a premedicant, it reduces the dose of subsequent anaesthetics and lengthens recovery.

Xylazine and medetomidine cause bradycardia (dogs' heart rates may fall to 40 beats/minute and cats to 70 beats/minute). Following intravenous injection, arterial blood pressure rises, then falls, stabilising at about 90% of the pre-sedation value. After intramuscular administration, the rise in pressure may not be seen. Respiration is depressed, and deeply sedated animals may show periods of up to 45 seconds' apnoea followed by a series of rapid breaths. Vomiting (more common in cats than dogs) may occur during the induction of sedation. These drugs have marked analgesic effects. They cause a cessation of gut motility, a rise in blood glucose, and increased urination through an increase in anti-diuretic hormone. When used as premedicants, they reduce the dose of subsequent anaesthetic required in a dose-related manner.

(c) Medetomidine and xylazine are alpha 2 adrenoceptor agonists, and their actions can be antagonised by alpha 2 adrenoceptor antagonists such as atipamezole or yohimbine.

106 (a) No. Advanced retinal degeneration of unknown aetiology.

(b) A complete absence of retinal blood vessels and increased tapetal reflectivity. Both eyes were equally affected and the animal was reported blind.

107 (a) The mass is the avulsed origin of the long digital extensor muscle. It changes position during flexion and extension of the joint.

(b) The mass usually appears as a calcified ovoid mass on the lateral aspect of the joint. A corresponding defect is sometimes seen in the lateral condyle of the femur.

(c) The treatment of choice is to re-attach the avulsed fragment with a lag screw and washer. If this is not possible, the bony fragment is excised and the tendon is sutured to the joint capsule or adjacent soft tissues in the most proximal position possible.

108 (a) Keratoconjunctivitis.

(b) Common predisposing causes include damage to the cornea by sharp items of bedding, projections in the cage, or (less frequently) fighting. Bacterial infections can then supervene.

109 There is a large mass in the chest, adjacent to the heart, which is likely to be a thymic lymphosarcoma or, rarely, a thymoma. The heart is not obviously enlarged, therefore other causes of murmurs such as anaemia or hypoproteinaemia should be considered.

110 (a) Acute ulcerative gingivitis (Vincent's disease).

(b) Usually, the lesion is teaming with spirochaetes.

(c) The drug of choice is metronidazole.

(d) The ulcerated gingival papillae will not regenerate and food stagnation in the spaces makes the re-occurence of the condition that much more likely. As with other forms of periodontal disease, there are genetic factors to this condition.

111 (a) A young animal with a history of poor growth suggests a congenital abnormality, and the other signs are consistent with hepatic or renal disease.
(b) In this case, a low blood urea (1.4 mmol/l) supports a diagnosis of a portovascular shunt, and the presence of a patent ductus venosus was confirmed by mesenteric venography. The episodes of profound lethargy and depression are associated with a high level of blood ammonia, which may be used diagnostically either as fasting levels or more usefully following protein intake.

The episodes of pyrexia are usually associated with bacteraemia which may result in foci of infections around the body, e.g. bone, kidneys. The radiography (*Figure 250*) follows the second injection of contrast into the mesenteric vein; the first injection is now seen as a pyelogram showing dilation of the renal pelvis. At post-mortem examination, ammonium urate calculi were discovered within the renal pelvises (*Figure 251*). Ammonium urate crystaluria is a frequent though intermittent finding in cases of porto-systemic shunting and may be useful diagnostically. The possibility of calculus disease, and the risk of urinary obstruction in males, should be borne in mind.

112 An extended ventro-dorsal view of the hips may be obtained under either general anaesthesia or moderate-to-heavy sedation. The dog is placed on its back, preferably supported in a trough to ensure stability. A sandbag placed over the sternum behind the elbows will secure the front end; the forelimbs may also be tied to hooks on the table edge if required. A looped tape is placed around each hind leg above the hock, the legs are extended and the tapes secured to hooks on the table end. A third tape is placed around the stifles to bring the femora parallel to each other and to ensure that the stifles are aligned in a cranio-caudal direction. The beam is centred on the cranial rim of the pubis.

If the cassette is placed in a cassette tunnel under the dog, the film may be removed and processed without disturbing the patient, allowing re-adjustment if the initial positioning is found to be imperfect.

113 (a) The evidence for the diagnosis of pyometra is purely circumstantial. There are a number of conditions which might cause the abnormalities seen in this case and, in the absence of positive evidence of a pyometra (vulval discharge or evidence of uterine enlargement), a definite diagnosis is thus premature.
(b) Other likely conditions include renal failure, diabetes mellitus and certain liver disorders (e.g. neoplasia). Hypercalcaemia is less common but could also produce these signs. Other causes of polydipsia such as Cushing's disease and diabetes insipidus are much less likely on the information available.
(c) To cover the likely possibilities, tests performed should include urea, creatinine, glucose, liver enyzmes (ALT + ALP), calcium, and perhaps total protein and albumin.
(d) The results of this group of tests clearly demonstrate that this is a case of diabetes mellitus. There is also evidence of hepatocellular damage, probably as a result of fatty infiltration of the liver.
(e) Neutrophilia (± monocytosis) is a common finding in animals with liver disease, due probably to a reduced resistance to infection, and is part of the fatty liver picture in this case. The same effect is often seen in neoplasia cases and in animals with chronic renal failure.
(f) This is a case of Type II diabetes, where the problem is insulin resistance rather than insulin deficiency. In these cases, high levels of an insulin antagonist lead to clinical diabetes mellitus, even in the presence of normal insulin secretion. In bitches a few weeks after oestrus this effect is caused by progesterone, and in susceptible animals can

lead to clinical signs very similar to those of pyometra at approximately the same time as a pyometra would be likely to occur.

(g) Spaying the bitch would be the best initial approach. This removes the source of the insulin antagonism and may in itself resolve the diabetes.

This bitch was spayed approximately 10 days after first presentation. The hyperglycaemia persisted, however, and a plasma insulin concentration of 5.6 mU/l was then demonstrated, indicating the development of an absolute insulin deficiency. Stabilisation on insulin was straightforward, though this would almost certainly not have been the case had the bitch been left entire, as the insulin antagonism effect would have been difficult to overcome.

114 (a) A bilateral plantigrade stance due to hyperextension of the carpi.

(b) Laxity of the flexor tendons.

(c) Ensure the dog is not overweight and encourage moderate exercise on a regular basis. External coaptation is contra-indicated. Variable improvement is obtained.

115 Condition Patient	Patient
1 Nasal neoplasia	BF
2 Soft palate hyperplasia	DE
3 Laryngeal paralysis	BF
4 Stenotic nares	DE
5 Tracheal collapse	AG
6 Glosso-epiglottic entrapment	DE

Nasal neoplasia typically arises in dogs over 6 years old, and animals with a meso- or dolicho-cephalic head conformation are most prone. Although obstructive dyspnoea may be seen, recurring epistaxis is the most common presenting sign. There is no sex predisposition.

Soft palate hyperplasia, stenotic nares and **glosso-epiglottic entrapment** are all components of the brachycephalic obstructive-airway syndrome. This is likely to produce symptoms in younger animals, typically in their first or second summers.

Laryngeal paralysis is a condition which tends to afflict dogs between 25– 35 kg bodyweight. Males are more prone than bitches by a ratio of 2:1. Labradors usually begin to show signs after 10 years of age but Afghan hounds may be afflicted significantly earlier.

Tracheal Collapse is a condition of toy breeds, and dogs with the disorder usually present with a persistent 'honking' cough. The condition can first cause concern over a wide age range, i.e. 1–8 years. No sex predisposition has been recognised.

The other dogs listed come from groups where there are no major causes of obstructive dyspnoea.

116 (a) The most significant feature of this case is gross hypercalcaemia, which at this level is almost certainly due to either primary hyperparathyroidism or primary pseudohyperparathyroidism.

(b) The diagnosis is neoplasia of some description. Primary hyperparathyroidism is due to an adenoma of the parathyroid gland producing excess PTH, primary pseudohyperparathyroidism to a neoplasm of an unrelated tissue believed to be producing 'parathyroid hormone-related substance' which has a similar effect. The likeliest contenders are lymphosarcoma (usually mediastinal), peri-anal adenocarcinoma, and mammary neoplasia.

(c) Subsequent investigation should centre on a physical and radiological search for the offending tumour.

(d) Hypercalceamia blocks the response of the collecting ducts to ADH, leading to an inability to concentrate the urine, polyuria, and hence polydipsia. Over a period of time, urinary excretory insufficiency tends to develop, especially if water intake is restricted, and plasma urea and creatinine increase.

Clinical examination of this patient revealed no mammary or peri-anal tumours, and there was no evidence of enlargement of the parathyroid gland. Thoracic radiography revealed a large mediastinal mass with dorsal displacement of the trachea. This was assumed to be a lymphosarcoma. Initial response to chemotherapy was excellent, with rapid regression of the tumour mass; however, regrowth was equally rapid and the bitch died within 8 weeks of the initial diagnosis. Post-mortem examination confirmed the lesion as a lymphosarcoma. The two superficial masses which prompted the initial complaint were indeed benign lipomas with no relation to the clinical problem other than the fact that an unobserved weight loss had caused them to become more prominent and hence appear to be enlarging.

117 (a) No. Collie eye anomaly.
(b) Choroidal hypoplasia adjacent to the optic disc on the left-hand side and atypical coloboma of the disc at 3 o'clock.

118 (a) Atropine is the drug most commonly used as an anticholinergic in cats and dogs. Glycopyrrolate, a more recent drug, does not cross the bloodbrain barrier, has no central effects, and may therefore be preferable to atropine, particularly in the cat. In human use it is said to cause less tachycardia than atropine, but this difference appears less evident in the dog.
(b) Opinion is divided as to the use of anticholinergics for the premedication of cats and dogs, some anaesthetists using them routinely while others give them only when required (e.g. should bradycardia occur). Anticholinergics will counteract the bradycardia caused by medetomidine or xylazine, but here again their use is controversial as it may lead to tachyarrhythmias. However, the use of anticholinergic premedication is essential if drugs – such as ether – which stimulate salivary and bronchial secretions are employed, or for any surgical procedure (e.g. ophthalmic) likely to trigger vagal bradycardia or cardiac arrest.

119 All except (d) and (g); Canine adenovirus 1 and distemper may cause kennel cough in partially immune animals, while the other three are broadly accepted as primary causes of kennel cough.

120 (a) Severe cardiomegaly, left- and right-sided, 3½-rib-spaces wide at the heart base. The lung fields are reasonably clear dorsally but there is increased density in the hilar area, suggesting the presence of pulmonary oedema; and there is a small amount of residual pleural fluid which is obscuring detail in the more ventral parts of the chest, including the line of the diaphragm. The cranial lung lobes appear dense also, but the forelimbs are not as far forward as they should be. Marked hepatomegaly is present.
(b) Dilated cardiomyopathy, best confirmed using ultrasound.
(c) Diuretics mainly. If renal function is reasonable, digoxin could be used with care. Angiotension-converting enzyme inhibitors are proving useful in some cases. Antiar-

rhythmic drugs are probably best avoided because of their negatively inotropic effects. Aspirin could be given twice weekly in case of aortic thromboembolism.

121 No. In the dog, ectopic ureters almost invariably enter the bladder wall at the normal site but then travel intramurally to open ectopically beyond the trigone (usually into the urethra or vagina). More information is gained by contrast radiographic techniques than laparotomy!

122 (a) The three main conditions under consideration in this case are idiopathic epilepsy, hypoglycaemia and hypocalcaemia. Hypocalcaemia is very unusual as a spontaneous occurrence in adult male dogs, but it would be unwise to omit it from consideration entirely. Anaemia and certain types of cardiac abnormality can cause peculiar fits/collapse, but it is very unlikely that no sign of these conditions would have been apparent on clinical examination.
(b) Obviously plasma glucose and calcium must be measured, together with haematology to check for the possibility of anaemia. It would also be useful to measure urea and creatinine, principally to pick up any signs of circulatory problems, and it is generally wise to include plasma proteins and liver enzymes in any diagnostic test panel, as a general screen.
(c) Hypoglycaemia is the obvious reason for the clinical signs in this case. When a glucose concentration of less than 2 mmol/l is demonstrated, hyperinsulinism is almost always the cause, generally pointing to an insulin-producing tumour of the β cells of the pancreas ('insulinoma').
(d) Plasma insulin measurement is the next step in diagnosis. However, it is not the insulin concentration itself which is diagnostic, but its ratio to plasma-glucose concentration. Therefore, a glucose measurement simultaneous with the insulin measurement is necessary, either by carrying out the insulin assay on the sample already to hand or by collecting a sample to repeat the glucose test at the same time as the follow-up sample is collected for insulin.

Fortunately, it was possible in this case to measure insulin on the sample already available, and the result was 26 mU/l. Although this would be a perfectly normal insulin level in a normal dog, post-prandially, it is grossly abnormal in association with a plasma-glucose concentration of 1.8 mmol/l. The ratio for the demonstration of hyperinsulinism is calculated from:

$$\frac{\text{Insulin (mU/l)} \times 100}{(\text{glucose (mmol/l)} \times 18) - 30}$$

In a normal animal, this should be less than 30. The ratio in this case however, was 1083, indicative of gross hyperinsulinism, and insulinoma was considered to be the diagnosis. An exploratory laparotomy was performed, with the dog on a dextrose saline drip throughout surgery to prevent a hypoglycaemic crisis; a lesion about 1 cm in diameter was identified in the pancreas, and this was resected. Immediate post-operative recovery was uneventful, but approximately 3 weeks later the hypoglycaemic episodes began to recur, again increasing in frequency, with a plasma glucose as low as 0.8 mmol/l measured on one occasion. It was considered probable that metastasis had occurred before the tumour had been removed, and due to his worsening clinical condition the dog was put to sleep.

123 Rare-earth phosphors have two main advantages over conventional calcium tungstate phospor. First, they absorb a greater proportion of X-ray photons; and, secondly, they are more efficient at converting these photons into light. Thus, rare-earth screens make better use of the available X-ray beam and produce more light without any reduction in image quality. The reduction in the amount of radiation required to produce radiographs comparable with those using calcium tungstate permits the use of shorter exposure times. This not only decreases movement blur and reduces both personnel and patient dosage, but also improves image quality and extends the capabilities of low-powered apparatus. The only possible disadvantage is that over-exposure is likely to occur when radiographing the lower limbs of cats and small dogs, particularly if the timer does not go below 0.1 second. Thus, one cassette fitted with calcium tungstate screens should be retained.

124 (a) The pencil has punctured the egg in two places.
(b) This is indicative of poor calcification and is often a sign of calcium depletion, especially in birds that are persistent egg-layers. This condition is common in cockatiels.

125 (a) Papules and pustules.
(b) Coagulase-positive *Staphylococcus intermedius*.
(c) Atopic dermatitis, flea-allergic dermatitis, food allergy, and recurrent false pregnancies.

126 (a) The likely injury, in the absence of a wound, is a spontaneous rupture of the gastrocnemius tendon. This generally occurs at the musculotendinous junction.
(b) The Achilles mechanism is damaged by the injury to the gastrocnemius tendon but the superficial digital flexor tendon is still intact. This causes a partially dropped hock and hyperflexed toes.
(c) Resection of the gastrocnemius tendon to restore its previous length. The tendon should be sutured with a locking loop or triple pulley tendon suture. Post-operatively, the hock joint should be immobilised in extension for 6 weeks.

127 (a) Pyometra should be considered as a primary diagnosis for the clinical signs given above. However, the additional information of inspiratory stridor and excessive skin folding points to the possibility that the animal is acromegalic. Progesterone-induced acromegaly following metoestrus or progestogen administration is the commonest form seen in the bitch. Clinical signs are the result of progestogenic stimulation of growth hormone secretion. This results principally in two effects: growth-promoting stimulates the proliferation of soft tissue, bone and cartilage, whilst the catabolic effects of growth hormone produce insulin antagonism and therefore carbohydrate intolerance (signs consistent with diabetes mellitus).
(b) Pyometra may be ruled out using ultrasound examination, radiography or a total white cell count, while metoestrus acromegaly may produce haematological changes of hyperglycaemia and mild anaemia. Therapy for metoestrus acromegaly is ovariectomy. It is likely that cases of suspected 'pyometra' which respond to ovariohysterectomy and yet have no uterine infection are cases of metoestrus acromegaly.

128 (a) The parasite is the egg of a trematode.
(b) Such parasites can be treated with an appropriate anthelmintic, but proper control necessitates breaking the life-cycle: the trematode needs a mollusc as an intermediate host.

129 (a) *Toxoplasma gondii* and *Neospora caninum*.
(b) Toxoplasmosis may be indicated by rising serum antibody titres using a direct agglutination test. Neosporosis is indicated by rising serum antibody titres using an indirect immunofluorescence assay.

(c) Treatment with sulphonamide pyrimethamine may eliminate the infections but there is often little clinical improvement.

130 (a) Ketamine may be given to the cat by intravenous, intramuscular or subcutaneous injection, or it can be squirted into the mouth (it is absorbed across mucous membranes) – although this last method is less reliable.

(b) Used alone, ketamine causes convulsions in the dog.

(c) Ketamine has been used in combination with a wide variety of tranquillisers and sedatives, of which the alpha 2 adrenoceptor agonists (xylazine and medetomidine) have proven the most effective in reducing – if not always eliminating the convulsions.

131 (a) The differential diagnosis of a purulent unilateral nasal discharge in a middle-aged dolichocephalic dog includes:

(i) Chronic intra-nasal foreign body.

(ii) Mycotic rhinitis.

(iii) Chronic idiopathic hyperplastic rhinitis.

(iv) Dental periapical suppuration.

(v) Intra-nasal neoplasia.

The Irish Wolfhound Rhinitis syndrome (IWRS) has not been included because afflicted dogs rarely survive beyond 2 years of age. Also, the IWRS, together with other forms of hyperplastic rhinitis, generally produces a profuse bilateral mucus-based discharge. Intra-nasal parasitism is now so rare that it can be discounted as a possibility in the United Kingdom, but isolated cases of nasal infestation by the mite, *Pneumonyssus caninum*, and the helminth, *Capillaria aerophilia*, have been reported in the U.S.A.

(b) Diagnostic procedures:

(i) External assessment including measurement of air flow at nostrils.

(ii) Forced nasal flush and examination of the washings.

(iii) Radiography.

(iv) Rhinoscopy.

(v) Serological testing for aspergillosis.

(vi) Exploratory surgery.

Procedures (ii), (iii), (iv) and (vi) are performed under general anaesthesia. The retrograde technique for nasal flushing is preferred. This depends upon the placement of a Foley catheter into the nasopharynx by way of the mouth. The balloon is inflated once the tip of the catheter has been placed around the back of the palate. The remainder of the pharynx is packed to absorb excess fluid. The washings are collected at the nares. After spinning down, the sediment is examined for fungal hyphae, foreign matter, tumour cells etc.

Effective rhinoscopy (*Figure 252*) depends upon the availability of suitable equipment. A forward-viewing arthroscope is ideal as it is sufficiently long for a complete inspection of the conchal surfaces through to the nasopharynx. A 4.2 mm instrument is suitable for large dogs, but for small dogs and for cats a 2.5 mm endoscope is required. Otoscopes are of no value to view beyond the nasal vestibule. A flexible fibreoptic gastroscope is the ideal instrument for retrograde rhinoscopy via the nasopharynx (*Figure 253*).

Swabbing of the nasal discharge for culture and sensitivity testing is notoriously inaccurate, to the point where the results are likely to be misleading – especially when mycotic agents are present.

Agar gel double-diffusion testing of serum from suspect cases is a very reliable technique for the diagnosis of intra-nasal aspergillosis, provided that a wide range of antigenic serotypes is used, and that the patient is not immunosuppressed by concurrent corticosteroid medication.

132 (a) Myositis of the masticatory muscles. Atrophy of the temporal and masseter muscles is evident. Most dogs present with this atrophic form of myositis, but occasionally the condition is preceded by a painful inflammatory myositis.

(b) Histological findings in the inflammatory form include severe necrosis of the muscle fibres, and an inflammatory exudate composed mainly of mononuclear cells (lymphocytes, plasma cells and macrophages) and a small number of neutrophils. The atrophic form is characterised by degeneration and atrophy of muscle fibres, and increased amounts of scar tissue.

(c) The aetiology is uncertain but it is possible that certain factors predispose the masticatory muscles to undergo myopathic change. An auto-immune basis has been suggested.

133 No! This is purely an anatomical finding. While it is a common abnormality in bitches with urethral sphincter mechanism incompetence and may be a factor predisposing to urine leakage in such cases, it can also be found in a small proportion of normal bitches.

134 (a) This is 'bumblefoot' (pododermatitis) – usually a staphylococcal infection of the ball of the foot.

(b) It can be treated by a combination of antimicrobial therapy, surgery, and improvements in management, e.g. better perching surfaces, regular clipping of claws (talons).

135 Though (a) and (c) are broadly correct, not all fits are preceded by a prodromal period, particularly as more fits are experienced. Ataxia is a not infrequent consequence of mysoline therapy in the short term but usually disappears as the dog adapts to the drug. Under no circumstances should therapy be stopped abruptly or fits may ensue. Rather, it should be reduced gradually and, if no fits occur over many months, can then be stopped altogether in some cases.

136 The method of choice is (c). The complications of cystotomy are fewer and less serious than those of urethrotomy, and this enables all calculi to be removed at once. If (c) is not possible because the urethral calculi cannot be returned to the bladder, (b) is the next-best alternative. Vesical calculi, remaining after (b), can be dissolved *in situ* or removed via a cystotomy after healing of the urethrotomy.

137 (a) Histiocytoma, mast cell tumour

(b) While the prognosis for histiocytoma is excellent, with most cases regressing spontaneously, that for mast cell tumours is guarded, the treatment for solitary localised tumours often involving radical excision.

(c) These are neoplastic histiocytes.

138 (a) Under the conditions usually found in a veterinary surgery, pulse rates for dogs range from 70–180 and for cats from 145–200. Rates may be lower in fit working dogs, or if the animal is very relaxed. Generally, the higher rates are found in the smaller animals.

(b) Tachycardia may be due to fear, or to pre-existing cardiac or pulmonary disease. Frightened animals should be calmed by quiet handling, and adequately premedicated before induction of anaesthesia.

139 (a) The mouse has a slight rectal prolapse.

(b) There are many possible causes but a common one is infestation with the mouse pinworm, *Syphacia obvelata*, the female of which lays its eggs around the perineum; as a result, there may be pruritus leading to a prolapse.

140 (a) Subaortic stenosis.

(b) Guarded in short term, poor long term. There is no satisfactory surgical treatment at present, and most cases collapse at exercise or may drop dead suddenly due to arrhythmias. If sudden death does not occur, left heart failure will develop eventually.

141 The most common reasons for the failure of a sedative drug to have the desired effect are:

(i) Wrong choice of drug for the animal concerned (e.g. expecting a phenothiazine drug alone to sedate a vicious dog).

(ii) Incorrect method of administration (e.g. perivascular, into fat deposits, etc.).

(iii) Inadequate time allowed for drug to work. The time required depends on the drug, the route of administration, and the state of excitement of the animal. It is always longer than the busy veterinary surgeon anticipates.

(iv) The animal is very 'excited' before administration of sedative. When this happens, there are times when no sedative is effective.

142 Regurgitation associated with complete or segmental megoesophagus is seen in (a), (b) and (e). Pyloric stenosis leads to vomiting, while in mandibular neuropraxia, damage to the mandibular branch of the trigeminal nerve leads to an inability on the part of the dog to retain food within the mouth or move it to the pharynx. A patent ductus arteriosis does not constrict the oesophagus but leads to a left-to-right shunt of blood.

143 (a) The retained upper primary canine has forced its permanent successor to erupt rostrally. The lack of space is guiding the lower canine into a palatal occlusion which will eventually cause severe trauma to the palatal mucosa.

(b) **Early** extraction of the primary tooth, as well as caudal digital pressure to the upper canine by the owner, can create adequate space for eruption and atraumatic occlusion of the lower canine.

144 The majority of bitches whelp 63 days after ovulation (64–66 days after the surge of luteinising hormone). Confusion over the length of pregnancy occurs since the bitch may have a fertile mating several days before or after ovulation. The apparent pregnancy length – the time from mating to whelping – may range from 58–70 days.

145 (a) The bird has its head on one side.

(b) Differential diagnoses include trauma, poisoning, viral infections and thiamine deficiency. The bird also has a supernumerary digit – not uncommon in this species.

146 (a) This dog is suffering from **gastric dilatation** which has now progressed to gastric **volvulus** (torsion).

(b) The immediate priorities for management of GDV include:

(i) **Decompression** of the gastric dilatation by oesophageal entubation, needle gastrostomy, or temporary surgical gastrostomy.

(ii) **Fluid therapy** to manage hypovolaemic shock caused by the effective loss of blood in the portal circulation.

Surgical correction of the volvulus is **not** an immediate priority.

(c) Dogs with gastric dilatation/volvulus (GDV) may be **either acidotic or alkalotic**. The acute gastric ischaemia gives rise to anaerobic metabolism which tends to cause acidotic changes, while the sequestration of acidic gastric content in the lumen tends to cause alkalosis. Never assume or treat changes of either type in GDV unless blood gas monitoring is available to confirm them.

(d) A definitive surgical correction of the volvulus should be considered **only once the dog's shock status has been stabilised**. In most cases it is several hours before surgery can be safely considered, and some clinicians prefer to delay surgery for as long as 24 hours provided temporary gastrostomy has been performed.

(e) The ventral surface of the abdominal contents is obscured by the omentum, indicating **a clockwise volvulus** of the stomach. The stomach should therefore be carefully derotated in an anti-clockwise direction.

(f) The fundic area of the stomach shows severe **ischaemic necrosis** due to ischaemic damage to the **short gastric vessels**. The options are:

(i) **Resection** of the devitalised tissue.

(ii) **Invagination** of the affected area by means of inverting sutures or staples.

This should then be followed by **gastropexy** to prevent further episodes of gastric dilatation and volvulus occurring.

(g) The more common long-term complications of GDV include:

(i) **Gastric perforation** leading to gross peritoneal contamination.

(ii) The development of **cardiac arrythmias** as the result of myocardial ischaemia. As many as 40% of dogs with GDV present with this complication, but it is a common post-operative problem, too.

147 (b) and (d). Contrary to popular belief, uraemia and peritonitis are not the major concerns in these cases. The most serious consequences of bladder rupture are hyperkalaemia and acidosis because of their effects on the heart. For this reason, induction of anaesthesia to repair the bladder before correction of these metabolic abnormalities may be fatal.

148 (a) Calcinosis circumscripta may develop within the lingual tissues of fast-growing dogs of any of the medium-to-large breeds. The lesions may be sufficiently superficial to be obviously white and granular, but others are diagnosed on the basis of palpation alone.

(b) The disorder will not resolve spontaneously, although nor will the lesions increase in size once maturity is reached. Resection is effective provided it is complete, but surgery is necessary only if the lesion produces mechanical interference with tongue mobility.

149 (a) The low urea and raised ALP point towards some sort of liver disorder, and in an animal of under about 18 months of age a patent ductus venosus (congenital porto-caval shunt) is probably the first consideration when a liver problem is suspected. The low urea is particularly suggestive in this context.

(b) The appropriate tests are plasma ammonia and dynamic bile acids (although in this case only the post-prandial bile acid concentration was measured).

(c) The high ammonia confirms hyperammonaemia as the cause of the clinical signs (particularly the CNS signs) and explains the low urea (hyperammonaemia is caused by a failure of conversion of ammonia to urea), but the zero post-feeding bile acid concentration rules out any sort of porto-systemic shunt as the underlying physical cause in this case. It is impossible for an animal with a porto-systemic shunt to have no bile acids in the peripheral circulation 2 hours after a meal.

(d) The only other possible cause of hyperammonaemia (in the presence of low urea – it does occur as an incidental finding accompanying gross uraemia) is a failure of the metabolism of the urea cycle, due to an inborn error of metabolism. Canine cases are rare and the condition is in consequence little studied, but in man deficiencies of carbamoyl phosphate synthase and ornithine carbamoyl transferase are recognised. Reconsideration of the routine results in this case reveals that the only indicator of a liver disorder other than those involved in the urea cycle was the raised ALP – significantly, albumin was not at all low and ALT was normal. It was this raised ALP, suggesting more widespread liver problems, which had led the provisional diagnosis towards porto-caval shunt in the first place, but with that theory disproved it was considered that the ALP value could be explained either by the age of the dog (actively growing bones produce higher ALP activity) or by enzyme induction in the disrupted hepatic metabolism, or both.

The option of performing portal angiography to settle the question of porto-caval shunts with physical as well as metabolic certainty was rejected in this case as the owner was reluctant to give permission for invasive diagnostic procedures, and it was decided to attempt medical treatment. A diet with small amounts of high quality protein was formulated (based on cottage cheese and rice) to reduce the amount of nitrogen excretion to a minimum. In human patients sodium benzoate (0.1 g/kg/day given in the late evening) has been hailed as a 'miracle cure'. This forms an alternative pathway bypassing the urea cycle and allows the ammonia to be metabolised to hippuric acid, which is excreted harmlessly. It is not known whether this effect occurs in the dog also, but it was decided to attempt sodium benzoate treatment in this case. Initial response has been very encouraging, with the dog having gained 4 kg in 3 weeks.

150 (a) Fracture of the mandibular symphysis of a cat.
(b) This fracture can be repaired with a single wire passed behind the canine teeth and tightened around the mandibles. If the wire is tightened ventral to the symphysis, the knot can be buried in the soft tissues.
(c) A broad spectrum antibiotic should be given for 10–14 days since some contamination is inevitable, and soft food recommended for 2–3 weeks. The wire can be removed after 4–5 weeks, or when healing is complete.

151 (a) Schiff-Sherington syndrome.
(b) The Schiff-Sherington syndrome occurs in sudden complete compression of the thoraco-lumbar spinal cord. It is not seen in incomplete, sub-acute or chronic spinal cord lesions. In this case, the cord compression is likely to be due to a fracture or fracture-luxation of the spine.
(c) There is paralysis of the muscles caudal to the lesion and analgesia of the skin. The level of the lesion can best be determined by locating the line of analgesia, or the level of the panniculus reflex cut-off. This level is usually caudal to the spinal cord lesion by one or two cord segments due to the caudal emergence of the spinal nerves from the intervertebral foramina.

152 (a) Naturally occurring or iatrogenic hyperadrenocorticism.
(b) An ACTH stimulation test will differentiate between naturally occurring and iatrogenic disease.

(c) Diabetes mellitus is a serious complication in cases of hyperadrenocorticism, suggested here by the raised glucose level in a fasted dog.

153 (a) No. Central progressive retinal atrophy.
(b) The presence of several brown pigment spots over the tapetal fundus.

154 (a) Scattered radiation is produced when the primary beam interacts with the tissues, table top, cassette, etc., to produce new X-ray photons which are of longer wavelength than those of the primary beam and which emerge from the area penetrated in all directions. This emerging radiation presents a safety hazard to persons close to the animal and results in blurring of the image produced in the film.
(b) Scattered radiation can be controlled by:
   (i) Close collimation of the primary beam to the area under investigation.
   (ii) Using as low a kV as possible, after taking all other exposure considerations into account. Scattered radiation produces more problems with high kV settings.
   (iii) The use of rare-earth intensifying screens, which are less responsive to low-energy scattered radiation than are conventional calcium tungstate screens.
   (iv) The use of a grid. A grid is usually recommended for tissues which are more than 10 cm in depth.
   (v) The use of lead rubber placed under the non-screen film or cassette to prevent back scatter.

155 (a) There is wet matted fur beneath the jaw. This is commonly termed 'slobbers'.
(b) The most common cause is malocclusions, but bacterial or mycotic stomatitis can also occur.

156 The likely diagnosis is spermatogenic arrest. The aetiology of this condition is not entirely clear, although it manifests as an auto-immune orchitis. Affected dogs are otherwise healthy and usually have no history of malaise. The age of onset is variable, but often as early as 18 months. The condition has been shown to be inherited in some breeds of dog. There is no therapy.
   Very occasionally, dogs may fail to ejaculate the second fraction during collection; Attempts should therefore be made to collect for a second time.

157 (a) The technique is 'bubble contrast' echocardiography. Saline or plasma expander is repeatedly shaken or passed through a needle in and out of the syringe to create a milky suspension of micro bubbles which is injected into a peripheral vein while recording an ultrasound image. The bubbles are removed by the lungs and therefore should not enter the left side of the heart, unless there is a communication and a pressure difference between the right and left sides. The technique is particularly useful for demonstrating right-to-left shunting congenital defects.
(b) In this case, there is right ventricular hypertrophy due to pulmonic stenosis, and bubbles are passing through an atrial septal defect.

158 (a) The left side is preferable since most female birds have only a functional left ovary and oviduct, and it is important during a laparotomy to be able to examine the gonads.
(b) Birds are good subjects for laparotomy and laparoscopy because the air sacs act as an insufflated chamber, facilitating examination of internal organs.

159 (a), (c), (e) and (f). Reflex dyssynergia is a lack of detrusor-urethral co-ordination so that the urethra fails to relax as the bladder contracts during micturition, leading to dysuria. It may be voluntary or involuntary and the former may respond to diazepam or dantrolene, while the latter may be treated with alpha-blockers such as phenoxybenzamine.

160 The tips of the lower canines have been worn down through attrition against the upper third incisors. The cause has been a malocclusion of the teeth. Occasionally, the teeth are not worn down or forced into an abnormal position but mobility and exfoliation of the teeth may occur through alveolar bone loss due to the traumatic bite.

161 Non-rebreathing circuits have the major advantage that the concentration of anaesthetic gases delivered from the machine is the concentration of gases that the animal breathes, making it easy to obtain stable anaesthesia. The circuits can be designed to have low dead space and low resistance. Inspiration of cold dry gases leads to loss of fluid and heat from the animal. Comparatively high flow rates are required, being expensive in gas, and leading to pollution of the operating environment.

Rebreathing circuits (i.e. those incorporating soda lime for absorption of carbon dioxide) require lower gas flows, and so can be more economical to run. Their use conserves heat and moisture in the circuit. Resistance in some (but not all) rebreathing circuits can be high. At low flow rates of fresh gas it is difficult to maintain adequate concentrations of volatile agents to ensure anaesthesia. 'In circle' vaporisers prevent this problem but can result in high anaesthetic concentrations. The major disadvantage with rebreathing systems is that, without expensive electronic monitoring equipment, it is impossible to know the concentration of anaesthetic gases, or of oxygen, in the circuit.

162 Sarcoptic mange, Cushing's disease, nutritional deficiencies/imbalances, and endocrinological disorders.

163 There are various differential diagnoses, including gapeworm (*Syngamus trachea* infestation) and bacterial tracheitis/pneumonia, but the most likely in a bird of prey with these signs is aspergillosis (*Aspergillus fumigatus* infection).

164 (a) Plantar subluxation of the proximal intertarsal joint.
(b) The subluxation is due to a rupture of the plantar ligament, or an avulsion of the ligament from its origin on the base of the calcaneus (os calcis).
(c) Arthrodesis of the calcaneo-quartal joint with a pin and figure-of-eight tension band wire.

165 The tongue is cyanotic at rest. The most likely diagnosis is tetralogy of Fallot, which is a multiple defect consisting of pulmonic stenosis, a ventricular septal defect, an overriding aorta, and right ventricular hypertrophy. Cyanosis on exertion only may suggest a less severe defect, e.g. pulmonic stenosis with an atrial or ventricular septal defect, or a large reverse-shunting septal defect alone.

166 It is the differential absorption of the X-ray beam that allows radiographic images of patients to be produced. X-ray absorption by a substance is affected by the effective atomic number of its elements and the physical density of the substance.

There are six perceptible degrees of tissue radiodensity: air, fat fluid/soft tissue, bone, positive-contrast media, and metal. These substances are increasingly radiopaque because of their increasing effective atomic number, except for air which has an effective atomic number similar to that of soft tissue but has a much lower physical density.

167 (a), (d), (e) and (f) are true: cats do not appear to be susceptible to **Leptospira** spp. and the organisms do not appear to play a part in renal disease in this species. Diagnosis in dogs is based on demonstration of the motile organisms in urine under dark field microscopy. The organisms are readily cultured from field cases. Serology, as a rising titre, may be valuable in retrospect.

168 (a) The lesion represents extensive calcinosis cutis and secondary bacterial dermatitis associated with hyperadrenocorticalism (Cushing's disease). The lethargy, polydypsia, good appetite and apparent increase in weight due to a pendulous abdomen are consistent with the diagnosis but the bitch does not show the classic alopecia that most associate with the condition. Calcinosis cutis is seen in about 20% of cases of Cushing's but is infrequently as striking as in this case.
(b) Confirmation of the diagnosis is by blood control measurements following ACTH stimulation or dexamethasone administration (high or low dose). Haematology and routine blood biochemistry show changes consistent with, but not diagnostic of, Cushing's syndrome.
   Treatment of this case, a pituitary hyperadrenocorticalism, with *op* DDD led to a resolution of the skin lesions and an improvement of the dog's demeanour (*Figure 254*).

169 (a) No. Generalised progressive retinal atrophy.
(b) Narrow retinal blood vessels and hyper-reflectivity of the tapetal fundus. The two eyes showed identical clinical signs.

170 (c) and (e). Prostatis may result in pain, but (unless abscessation has occurred) the gland is usually symmetrical. Conversely, prostatic cysts result in asymmetry but are usually painless.

171 (a) Partial division of a single tooth bud which may be caused by physical trauma transmitted through the primary predecessor, or gemination – fusion of two separate tooth germs – which can be a heritable condition.
(b) The only significance of the condition is to 'show people', to whom the suggestion of congenitally absent teeth can be very important. A tooth count should confirm whether the condition is a true gemination or a partial division of a single bud.

172   When it is necessary to keep semen for only short periods of time (up to 3 days) it may be diluted in a milk extender, cooled and stored at about 4°C. Pasteurised milk boiled for 1 minute and then cooled should be used. The sperm-rich (second) fraction of the ejaculate should be diluted approximately 1:5 (volume/volume) with the extender at 37 °C. This is then placed in a polystyrene test tube lagged with cotton wool, and allowed to cool to room temperature. Following this (*Figures 255* and *256*), the test tube is placed in a second container, which is sealed and placed with ice cubes in an insulated flask. Two containers are required to allow the semen to cool slowly but to prevent it from freezing. Once packed like this the semen may remain viable for up to 5 days, although it is better used within 3 days. When it is required for use it can be inseminated immediately.

173 (a) The skin (including the spines) has been severely lacerated. Grass-cutting machines are a common cause of such damage.

(b) In recent cases suturing is feasible, under anaesthesia, but this laceration was inflicted several days previously and is best treated by débridement and regular irrigation, with a view to encouraging granulation. It is particularly important to prevent infestation by dipterous larvae (myiasis).

174 (a) Dermatophytosis caused by *Trichophyton erinacei*.

(b) Skin scrapings or fungal culture of stratum corneum.

(c) The Jack Russell terrier.

(d) Guarded – lengthy systemic treatment is often needed and cure may not be possible.

175 Topical administration of enilconazole through catheters implanted into the frontal sinuses. Each catheter is placed through a trephine hole into the caudal third of the sinus and secured by adhesive-tape 'butterflies' sutured to the skin (*Figure 257*). An Elizabethan collar is required to protect the catheter for the duration of the treatment, which is usually completed within 7–12 days. Bilateral treatment is advocated for all cases where there are the slightest grounds to suspect that the mycosis may have extended to the contralateral side.

Enilconazole is administered twice daily at a dose rate of 10 mg/kg diluted in saline to a total volume of 5–10 ml. The frontal sinuses act as header tanks for the medication to pass into the nasal chambers. The treatment is continued until the nasal washings are clear and the discharge has resolved. Rhinoscopy is repeated to confirm elimination of the mycosis before the catheters are removed.

Systemic antimycotic medication with agents such as thiabendazole or ketoconazole is no longer regarded as necessary or even desirable as these agents can be hepatotoxic.

176 Non-screen film is X-ray film used without the benefit of an intensifying screen. The radiographic image is therefore entirely due to X-ray photons, rather than to visible light produced by screens.

Advantages

(i) Extremely fine radiographic detail, as there is no 'screen unsharpness'.

(ii) Small size of film allows placement in mouth for intra-oral work.

Disadvantages

(i) Increased exposure required: the mAs factor must be increased by about 25–50 times compared with screen film used in a cassette. As this usually means the use of a long exposure time, the patient must be anaesthetised.

(ii) Greater radiation risk to the patient due to increased exposure (N.B. under no circumstances should animals be held for exposures using non-screen film).

(iii) Thicker emulsion requires slightly longer developing, fixing and drying times. This may make some non-screen film unsuitable for automatic processing.

(iv) Envelope wrapping renders film more susceptible to crimping or bite marks from lightly anaesthetised patients.

In practice, non-screen film is used almost exclusively for intra-oral work (but occasionally for radiographs of digits or of small exotic animals).

177 Differential diagnoses include fight wounds, ectromelia (mouse pox) and ecto-parasites. The involvement of both sexes would tend to exclude fighting. The lesions are not typical of ectromelia in that the feet and tail are not involved. Infestation with *Myobia musculi* is most likely; the mites can usually be seen with a handlens.

178 (c), (d) and (e) are true. Clinical signs of tracheal collapse may not be seen until middle-age in some animals, although the predisposition is present from birth. Brachycephalics are not seemingly predisposed, the condition occurring primarily in toy breeds such as the Yorkshire terrier. Diagnosis is rarely possible on plain radiographs, and even fluoroscopy may not be helpful. History, breed and clinical signs are usually suggestive; bronchoscopy is frequently helpful, though the management of anaesthesia may present problems.

179 (a) That of non-selective angiography. Radiographs obtained following the rapid injection of a contrast medium (iohexol) into a peripheral vein, are exposed at frequent time intervals to reveal contrast filling of the right and left sides of the heart (*Figures 133* and *134*).
(b) The left side of the heart (*Figure 134*) is normal, but the right side (*133*) shows hypertrophy of the ventricle wall, narrowing (stenosis) in the region of the pulmonary valve, and a post-stenotic dilation.

180 (a) Atopic dermatitis.
(b) An intra-dermal test with likely allergens. This is not specific, however, and other allergic dermatoses should always be ruled out.
(c) Management of atopic dermatitis involves either avoiding the allergen(s) involved, desensitisation, or more usually anti-inflammatory treatment. Concern about the dangers of steroid side-effects has recently led to the development of essential fatty acid therapy in cases of atopy.

181 (a) Yes.
(b) Good retinal blood supply with an absence of tapetum and areas of subalbinism in the non-tapetal fundus, the latter also associated with an heterochromic iris and the merle coat colour.

182 (a) This is a proliferative lesion. The likely cause is trauma due to a rough substrate.
(b) The best method of treatment would probably be cryotherapy. Attention needs to be paid to the environment.

183 (a) A close-fitting custom-formed acrylic plate covering the hard palate and wired to the primary teeth will offer excellent immobilisation and healing in 2–3 weeks. It is important to cure the material out of the mouth to avoid chemical and thermal burns that may occur while the material is setting.
(b) Injury to the alveolus may result in damage to the vascular supply of the developing and unerupted permanent teeth in the fracture line. It is important to check regularly on the eruption of these teeth after healing of the fracture and to extract any which are erupting non-vital and infected.

184 The 'praying' position is classically adopted by dogs with chronic anterior abdominal pain. This condition may be associated with a variety of causes, including chronic pancreatitis, gastric or duodenal ulceration, and, in older dogs, neoplasia within the anterior abdomen. In this dog, the intermittent vomition and the chronic and continuous nature of the condition in the absence of depression or progression of signs are suggestive of a chronic partial obstruction of the intestine. A fabric foreign body was removed from the stomach and duodenum, and the dog made an uneventful recovery.

185 A ball or similar foreign body lodged in the pharynx of a dog can cause rapid and fatal asphyxiation unless the owner can remove it quickly. Homes with solid-fuel fires may have coal tongs available and these are ideal for the withdrawal of large objects from the pharynx. When a hollow ball,i.e. a tennis ball, is involved, a stab into the ball followed by the application of a corkscrew action is an alternative possibility.

186 (a) No. Optic neuritis.
(b) A swollen optic disc with congestion of retinal blood vessels on the disc. The presenting signs were sudden blindness; the condition was bilateral, the pupils were widely dilated and there was no pupillary light reflex.

187 (a) Neuromuscular blocking agents give profound relaxation, greatly improving surgical conditions for a wide variety of surgical procedures, particularly in the dog. In the cat their major use is to prevent laryngeal spasm at intubation. As it becomes no longer necessary to use high doses of general anaesthetic agents for relaxation, cardiovascular parameters are better maintained. However, **it is essential to ensure that the animal is unconscious.** Once a neuromuscular blocking agent has been given, breathing is abolished (artificial ventilation is necessary), all somatic muscles are paralysed, and the usual signs of anaesthesia are no longer evident.
(b) The depth of anaesthesia can be judged by:

(i) The pulse rate. If this rises in response to a painful stimulus, analgesia is inadequate. However, appreciation of pain will occasionally cause a vaso-vagal reaction and brady-cardia results.

(ii) Pupil size. As the dog's eyes are now central the pupils are easily seen. The pupils dilate when anaesthesia is too light, constrict as it becomes adequate, then dilate again in deep anaesthesia. The use of atropine as a premedicant does not mask these changes in the dog, although it may do so in the cat.

(iii) Lacrymation will occur if analgesia is inadequate.

(iv) Except at maximal levels of neuromuscular blockade, the tongue may twitch slightly in response to pain. The presence of such a tongue twitch indicates the necessity for further analgesia, but its absence cannot be taken to mean that analgesia is adequate.

188 For the dog, the intra-oral occlusal view (film in mouth) using high-definition film is the single most informative projection in most instances as it is very effective for the evaluation of the turbinate tissues (*Figures 258* and *259*). This view permits the identification of areas of lysis of increased density, and the comparison of the two nasal chambers for asymmetry. The maxillary tooth roots, too, may be examined for periapical rarifaction. The frontal sinuses are best seen on the rostro-caudal skyline projection (*Figures 260* and *261*), which allows the two sides to be compared, and is helpful to establish whether intra-nasal disease has extended into the sinuses, i.e. in cases of aspergillosis or neoplasia. The lateral view is not generally recommended, first because it is less easy to interpret, and, secondly, since it rarely provides information not already identified on the other projections. Also, nasopharyngeal disorders are uncommon in dogs.

The intra-oral occlusal view is recommended for the cat, too; however, the skull conformation here renders the rostro-caudal skyline view of the frontal sinuses impracticable, although the latter can be seen well on the whole skull dorso-ventral projection. The lateral view of the head is likely to be more rewarding in the case of the cat because nasopharyngeal conditions such as polyps are not infrequent (*Figure 262*).

189 (a) The whiskers and hair around the snout are missing.
(b) This is 'barbering' due to plucking of the hairs by another mouse. Weight is added to the diagnosis by the fact that the lesions are bilaterally symmetrical.
(c) Confirmation is by careful observation and examination of the mice: the animal carrying out the barbering is usually the only one in the group with intact whiskers and hair!

190 (a), (c), (e) and (f) are true, (b) is **not**: infection in the cat, usually as a kitten, is followed by excretion of oocysts in vast numbers for about 3 weeks. Re-excretion after this is very uncommon. Also incorrect is (d); indeed, it is likely that most human infections are the result of ingestion of cysts in raw or undercooked meats. *Toxoplasma gondii* was described by Claude Nicol, in 1908 in Libya, in the muscle of the small rodent, the gondi.

191 (a) Examination of the distal tips of hairs often reveals evidence of self- trauma.
(b) Fleabite hypersensitivity, food hypersensitivity, and psychogenic alopecia.
(c) A circulating eosinophilia is a pointer towards allergic skin disease.

192 (a) This is the Northern mite (*Ornithonyssus sylviarum*).
(b) It is a significant parasite of birds since it sucks blood and can cause severe anaemia. However, it is often easier to detect than the red mite (*Dermanyssus gallinae*) because it completes its life-cycle on the host.

193 (a) The whole film, including the subject and the space between the two projections, is too dark. This is due to 'fogging' (darkening of the film not associated with the primary beam).
(b) There are several possible causes:
   (i) Light fogging due to improper storage and light leaking into the film box or hopper. This is unlikely in this case as the darkening is very diffuse rather than affecting one edge.
   (ii) Light fogging during processing, due either to the use of an incorrect safe light or white light entering the darkroom through chinks around the door. This is the most likely cause in practice.
   (iii) Storage fogging due to prolonged storage, or storage near chemical fumes or scattered radiation.
One other possibility is overdevelopment, due either to the use of developer which is too hot or the film being left in the developer for too long. Overdevelopment is unlikely in this case, however, since the background of each image is actually slightly **under-**developed.

194 (a) Lateral luxation of the elbow. Most luxations are lateral since the medial humeral condyle is larger than its lateral counterpart.
(b) The medial and lateral collateral ligaments. The joint is further stabilised by the interlocking of the anconeal process into the olecranon fossa.
(c) The extent of collateral ligament stability can be assessed by flexing the elbow and carpus to 90° and then rotating the foot. If the collateral ligaments are intact, only 45° of lateral rotation and 70° of medial rotation are possible. If the lateral ligament is served, the foot can be rotated 140° medially, while 90° of lateral rotation is possible with a ruptured medial collateral ligament.

195 (a) The radiographs (*Figure 147* and *148*) show 'microcardia' with a narrow caudal vena cava, suggesting severe hypovolaemia.

(b) Plasma electrolytes (particularly potassium) and plasma urea/creatinine and urine specific gravity. The signs are suspicious of hypoadrenocorticism but could be confused with acute renal failure. A cortisol level and ACTH stimulation test could be performed once fluid therapy has been started.

196 (a) Yes.

(b) Excellent retinal blood supply over a sparsely scattered tapetal fundus with a normal optic disk.

197 (a) Canine Wobbler syndrome.

(b) In the middle-aged Dobermann the likely cause of cervical spinal cord compression is disk degeneration secondary to cervical vertebral instability. Hypertrophy of the dorsal longitudinal ligament and degenerative changes involving the articular facets may also contribute to the cord compression.

(c) Establish the exact cause of cord compression with plain and contrast radiography. Myelograms of the neck in a neutral, flexed and extended position, as well as a traction view, are indicated. Mild cases may be managed conservatively. Surgery may involve decompression of the cord with a ventral slot procedure or distraction and arthrodesis of affected intervertebral joints with one of several techniques that are available.

198 (a) The synovial sarcoma is the most common articular tumour. Less frequently, tumours invade joints from extra-synovial sites, and only rarely metastasise to a joint.

(b) Soft tissue swelling in the early stages, progressing to destruction of the bones of the joint.

(c) The prognosis is poor. The tumour metastasises to the regional lymph nodes and the lungs.

199 (a) The condition is known as chronic gingivitis/stomatitis and the aetiology is unclear.

(b) It is known to be associated in many cases with persistent calicivirus and feline immunodeficiency infection. There is frequently secondary bacterial infection. A minority of cases of stomatitis are associated with chronic renal failure, diabetes mellitus and, rarely, hypervitaminosis A, and these should be eliminated as causes. Biopsy of the lesions shows chronic inflammatory reaction characterised typically by plasma cell and lymphocytic infiltration.

(c) Teeth cleaning, removal of exuberant tissue, and treatment with antibiotics such as metronidazole and ampicillin, may provide temporary improvement − but recurrence invariably occurs. Corticosteroids provide some relief but continuous therapy is necessary and is almost certainly not influencing the underlying cause.

200 (a) The smaller the animal, the more likely is hypothermia to occur during anaesthesia. It is a particularly severe problem for birds and small mammals, but can occur in any cat or dog, especially if anaesthesia is prolonged, or the chest or abdominal cavities are open for a length of time.

(b) Heat loss may be reduced by having a high temperature in the operating theatre, by minimal clipping of fur and hair, and by minimal wetting, particularly with agents such as spirit. Animals may be wrapped in foil, or bubble polythene, to conserve heat, and placed on a heated pad (care must be taken not to overheat). Where the animal is of suitable size the use of rebreathing anaesthetic circuits (i.e. with soda lime) conserves heat and moisture.

201 (a) Underdevelopment – i.e. background grey not black.
(b) There are numerous extraneous white and grey marks on the film, representing dirt and dried-on splashes on the intensifying screens. The screens should be cleaned regularly using cotton wool and a proprietary cleaner or mild soap.
(c) Some of the larger marks may be due to splashes onto the film itself before development. This can be rectified by separating the dry and wet areas within the darkroom and by careful handling of the film during processing.

202 (a) No. Plain radiographs are no better than 20% accurate in the diagnosis of tracheal collapse. The condition is dynamic and the possibility of an exposure being made at the moment of maximum collapse is slight.
(b) No. Although in theory fluoroscopy should be useful to capture the variations of tracheal diameter through the respiratory cycle, it is effective only if dynamic collapse occurs during the period of the examination. Accuracy levels a little over 50% are claimed.
(c) Yes. Provided suitable equipment is available, endoscopy is the best technique to diagnose tracheal collapse in the dog. The suspect patient is likely to be a toy dog and, therefore, the diameter of the endoscope should not exceed 4.5 mm if any room for respiration is to be left. Endoscopy affords the means to inspect the lumen of the trachea throughout its length to the carina, and also permits an assessment of laryngeal function. The endoscopic view in *Figure 263* came from a 4-year-old Yorkshire terrier with Grade 4 (out of 5) collapse.

203 (a) Primary glaucoma.
(b) Enlargement of the globe, congestion of conjunctival vessels, fractures in Descemet's membrane (vertical and horizontal grey lines) and ventral luxation of the lens with consequent aphakic crescent.

204 (a) The dog's symptoms are consistent with an episode of **hepatic encephalopathy**. In a dog of this age **porto-systemic shunting** is a likely cause of the encephalopathy. The dog's neurological signs should be managed by:
  (i) **Withdrawing all protein** food.
  (ii) Administering **enemas** to sterilise the bowel microflora (iodine, lactulose).
  (iii) **Fluid therapy** using Ringer's solution with dextrose and potassium, but avoiding lactated or acetated fluids which require hepatic conversion to bicarbonate.
  (iv) **Gut-active antibiotics**, to reduce bowel microflora.
  (v) The avoidance of sedatives and barbiturates if at all possible because of their prolonged hepatic metabolism. Diazepam may be used in cases of severe neurological dysfunction.
(b) Additional tests include **BSP retention** and **pre-and post-prandial bile salt** studies to confirm the presence of impaired hepatic metabolism.

(c) Venography shows the contrast reaching the heart without highlighting the portal circulation of the liver. The study confirms **gastrosplenic shunting of portal blood** into the caudal vena cava.

(d) The **shunt** should be isolated and **ligated** at laparotomy. The portal and central venous blood pressure should be monitored during surgery and ligation performed without increasing the portal pressure above 20 cm of water.

(e) The post-operative portogram demonstrates that the **shunt has been ligated** and there is now a normal portal blood circulation in the liver.

(f) Hypovolaemia in the post-operative period most often indicates **portal hypertension** caused by over-ligation of the shunt. Following stabilisation of the shock, surgery should again be performed to allow **the ligature to be loosened or even temporarily removed**.

205 (a) Contracture of the infraspinatus muscle.

(b) The limb is abducted on flexion of the shoulder. No change in posture is seen on shoulder extension.

(c) Degeneration, atrophy and fibrosis of the muscle fibres.

206 (a) The radiograph (*Figure 159*) shows evidence of emphysematous cystitis. The bladder is reasonably well distended, but has a greatly thickened irregular wall whose 'flaky pastry' appearance betrays the presence of layers of gas trapped within. This type of cystitis is an uncommon complication of diabetes mellitus and is associated with lower urinary tract infection with gas-forming organisms, such as *Proteus* or *E. coli*, which ferment the urinary glucose. Emphysematous cystitis can often be appreciated on palpation as a 'crackling' sensation in the caudal abdomen.

(b) Urine analysis and culture are indicated to establish the presence of glycosuria and provide a sensitivity for the necessary vigorous therapy. Blood glucose ($\pm$ blood insulin levels) is necessary to confirm diabetes mellitus, classically seen in middle-aged entire bitches, and to rule out other, rare, courses of glycosuria. Management of diabetes mellitus can then be initiated.

207 (a) Generalised demodicosis.

(b) In thickened scarred skin of severe cases scrapings are sometimes negative. In such cases, examination of purulent material from pustules and bullae is often more rewarding.

(c) Topical miticidal dips (amitraz or rotenone) are the most effective treatments, used in conjunction with topical and parenteral antibiosis.

(d) The prognosis is guarded in generalised cases of demodicosis; however, most can be controlled if not cured with the therapy suggested.

(e) Generalised demodicosis is considered an inherited disease and thus the owner must be advised **not** to breed from this dog.

208 (a) A sudden onset of a spontaneous bleeding problem in an adult dog with no previous history of bleeding episodes is nearly always related to either warfarin poisoning or thrombocytopenia. Congenital coagulopathies very seldom appear out of the blue in an adult patient. The gender of the dog rules out such sex-linked recessives as haemophilia A and Christmas disease, which occur clinically in males only.

(b) Warfarin poisoning is ruled out by the normal prothrombin time, and the extreme scarcity of platelets on the blood film confirms thrombocytopenia as the cause of the bleeding problem.

(c) The blood picture also shows a very marked granulocytopenia, and an anaemia which is non-regenerative in spite of the known blood loss. This indicates general bone marrow failure as opposed to any condition confined to the platelets.

(d) A marrow biopsy is necessary to confirm this, both by the failure to find haemopoietic marrow where it ought to be and by a very acellular appearance in any marrow harvested. However, this procedure should be undertaken with caution in a severely thrombocytopenic patient.

(e) Although many cases of bone marrow aplasia are spontaneous, many others are a result of an adverse drug reaction. The most common drugs implicated in these occurrences are the oestrogens, and in fact this bitch had been given an injection of oestradiol benzoate for a misalliance during oestrus 2 weeks earlier. It is highly probable that this was the cause of the bone marrow aplasia in this case.

(f) The prognosis is poor. Occasionally, bone marrow function does return in such cases, but in most cases it does not. The severe neutropenia and totally non-regenerative red cell picture in this instance are not encouraging signs.

It was considered that the diagnosis in this case was sufficiently definite for a bone marrow biopsy to be omitted. Treatment was begun with testosterone and anabolic steroids in the hope of encouraging the bone marrow back into activity, and with antibiotic cover to counteract the pyrexia caused by the neutropenia. The neutrophil count stabilised at about 1×10^9/l, the pyrexia abated, and although platelets remained scarce the petechiation and haemorrhage gradually ceased. However, PCV continued to decline despite the cessation of blood loss, and the bitch became progressively weaker and intolerant of exercise. A blood transfusion produced a temporary improvement, but the anaemia again worsened steadily and the patient was put to sleep with a PCV of 0.07. At post-mortem examination there was only a tiny amount of red marrow in the centre of the femurs, with most of the marrow space containing only fat.

209 The left nasal chamber (on the right of the radiograph in *Figure 162*) shows extensive turbinate bone destruction with replacement by a diffuse increase in density. There is a circumscribed area centrally which is slightly less radiodense and this represents destruction of the overlying hard palate or maxilla. The composite shadow of the vomer bone and the cartilaginous nasal septum normally seen in the midline is largely destroyed. The right nasal chamber is normal.

Diagnosis: left-sided malignant nasal tumour.

210 (a) The lateral chest X-ray (*Figure 164*) clearly shows an enormous cardiac silhouette due to pericardial disease. Although peritoneopericardial diaphragmatic hernias are recorded in dogs, the likeliest diagnosis in a St. Bernard is idiopathic pericardial effusion. In this condition a large volume of sterile bloody fluid collects in the pericardial sac, causing compression of the heart and signs of right-sided cardiac failure.

(b) *Figure 163's* ECG shows sinus tachycardia and low-voltage QRS complexes. Right bundle branch block (RBBB) is present. The ECG in *Figure 165* shows that, after fluid drainage, the heart rate is normal, but that low-voltage QRS complexes and RBBB are still present. The P waves are prolonged. Underlying heart disease is a possibility.

211 (a) Prolapse of the vagina and bladder eversion.

(b) By gentle lavage with non-irritant solution (e.g. normal saline), reduction, and the use of a purse-string suture in the vulva. It is important to determine and correct the cause of tenesmus (e.g. dystokia, cystitis or, as in this case, severe vaginitis).

212 (a) An oro-nasal fistula may be a sequel to long-standing periodontal disease where the thin medial bony wall of the upper canine socket has been destroyed by chronic infection. The defect can also be created through the extraction of the upper canine.

(b) Predictable repair of the fistula depends on:
  (i) Thorough débridement of the area of all infected material.
  (ii) Freshening up the margins of the fistula.
  (iii) A flap closure free of tension.

213 (a) The left ureter contains a blood clot (hence the renal pelvic and proximal ureteral dilatations – because of partial outflow obstruction from the left kidney – and the vermiform filling defects detected radiographically in the bladder).

(b) This suggests renal bleeding which may be idiopathic, traumatic or neoplastic in origin. Trauma severe enough to cause this degree of haemorrhage would have resulted in detectable radiographic abnormalities of the kidney and is unlikely to have persisted for this length of time. The likely diagnoses, therefore, are idiopathic renal haemorrhage or renal neoplasia. Although the latter was not detectable grossly on clinical and radiographic investigations and observation (*Figure 169*), minute renal haemangiomas or haemangiosarcomas can result in profuse haematuria, and yet be difficult to detect except on histopathological examinations.

(c) The surgical treatment, assuming a normal second kidney is present and there is no evidence of metastases, is left nephrectomy.

214 (a) Synchysis scintillans (numerous reflective particles moving within a fluid vitreous).

(b) Retinal degeneration.

215 (a) The combination in an older cat, of weight loss, increased appetite, and diarrhoea, is strongly suggestive of hyperthyroidism.

(b) Clinical examination may reveal uni-or bilateral enlargement of the thyroid glands, though these are not always palpable and occasionally ectopic thyroid tissue may be involved. Tachycardia (<180 b/m) is invariably present and, depending upon the degree of secondary cardiomyopathy, there may be a systolic murmur and/or a degree of congestive heart failure with tachypnoea or dyspnoea.

(c) Diagnosis may be confirmed by the demonstration of resting T4 levels; a stimulation test is not always necessary. The major differential diagnoses, chronic renal failure and intestinal lymphosarcoma, are usually associated with decreased appetite and depression. Diabetes mellitus is less common and may be eliminated by routine biochemistry.

216 (a) Auscultation is taken place through a towel. This method has much to commend it as the towel reduces extraneous sounds, including scratching on the animal's 'shell' (carapace).

(b) As in mammals, auscultation can assist in the diagnosis of respiratory infections, cardiac disease, and certain alimentary tract disorders.

217 (a) Cryptorchidism is the most likely diagnosis; monorchidism is extremely rare.

(b) Cryptorchidism is believed to be a sex-linked autosomal recessive trait. There is a significant breed predisposition, and the owner should be advised not to breed from affected animals and/or their parents (which are carriers).

(c) Medical therapy for cryptorchidism is not usually successful and is unethical. Because of the increased risk of testicular neoplasia and testicular torsion in the abdominal testis and because of the genetic predisposition, both the retained and the scrotal testes should be removed (*Figures 264–266*). Occasionally, ectopic testes are found to have passed through the inguinal canal but not to have entered the scrotum.

218 (a)The indications for partial laryngectomy – excision of the tissues which intrude into the laryngeal airway – include:
 (i) Debarking.
 (ii) Chondritis.
 (iii) Paralysis.
 (iv) Neoplasia.
Partial laryngectomy can be performed per os or by ventral laryngofissure, but in either case a bypass tracheotomy is needed to provide for anaesthetic maintenance and post-operative care. The tissues removed may include the true and false vocal folds, the vocal process of the arytenoid cartilage, and the ventral projection of the cuneiform appendage. Partial laryngectomy offers the only treatment option, short of total laryngectomy, for the removal of chronically infected cartilage or neoplastic tissue from the larynx.
(b) The complication which arose is known as laryngeal 'webbing' and consists of excessive fibrosis and granulation tissue at sites which were denuded in the surgery. There is a higher risk of this complication when the procedure is performed to treat laryngeal paralysis, but it can occur regardless of the original indication. This is a major reason why the technique should be abandoned as a treatment for paralysis in favour of one of the safer and more effective methods, such as arytenoid lateralisation or prosthetic laryngoplasty.
 Figures 173 and *174* serve as a warning that debarking is not without serious risk of major complication and should be avoided if at all possible.

219 (a) These are abscesses. Investigations should consist of observation and examination of the animals and needle aspiration of material from the lesions. Aspiration reveals polymorphs and bacteria, usually staphylococci.
(b) Prevention is best achieved by isolation of affected animals, by minimising fighting, and by careful attention to hygiene.

220 With the head positioned in semi-flexion, the axis is seen to be subluxated with respect to the atlas, such that the two vertebrae are no longer aligned, but instead form an angle of about 140°. The inter-vertebral foramen (between the neural arch of C1 and the spinous process of C2) is greatly widened. In this instance, the cause is aplasia of the odontoid peg of the axis; the cranial end of the body of the axis is clearly seen and lacks the normal cranial extension which represents the peg.
 Diagnosis: atlanto-axial subluxation due to aplasia of the odontoid peg.

221 (a) The radiograph (*Figure 177*) shows a (normal) bilobed swim bladder. There are stones in the stomach which may or may not be normal.
(b) The prominent teeth are a feature of this species!

222 (a) The radiograph shows a pathological fracture of the mandible secondary to chronic periodontal disease which has destroyed a considerable amount of alveolar bone.

(b) The immediate treatment is to extract the teeth in the fracture line, thoroughly debride to healthy bone, repair the soft tissue defect, and commence an aggressive regime of antibiotic treatment. Fibrous healing will usually result. The shift in the position of the mandible may cause trauma to the palate from the lower canine of the opposite side. This should be shortened and root-filled if necessary.

223 (a) Solar dermatitis (actinic keratosis).
(b) Either by the application of topical sunscreens, by the avoidance of direct sunlight, or by surgical resection of the pinnal margin.
(c) Squamous cell carcinoma.

224 (a) It is probable that there is an oestrous bitch in the neighbourhood; pheromones may travel long distances, so that the 'culprit' may not be immediately obvious. Not all male dogs attempt to 'escape' in these circumstances, especially if they are unaccustomed to going out other than in human company.
(b) Short-term treatment is usually with progestogens. Delmadinone acetate or medroxyprogesterone acetate may be given subcutaneously, or megestrol acetate may be administered orally. Sedatives may also be useful (e.g. acetylpromazine). Orchidectomy should be considered for long-term therapy, although it may not be immediately effective in adult dogs.

225 (a) Ventricular premature complexes may be due to primary heart disease, secondary to non-cardiac disease, or to drug treatment – but often the cause is impossible to determine. A thorough clinical and cardiological work-up is advisable, therefore. If no abnormalities are found in an asymptomatic dog, no treatment is required. (However, many authors suggest that therapy should be given if more than 15 ectopics per minute are present on the ECG.)
(b) Regular monitoring in case cardiac disease develops, and immediate re-examination if the dog becomes unwilling to exercise.

226 (a) This is clearly a case of acute leukaemia.
(b) RBC picture is normal, platelets appear scarce/adequate. Although the blood film is overrun with lymphocytes, crowding out all other white cell types, morphology of the lymphocytes is essentially normal, with no prolymphocytes, lymphoblasts or bizarre cells visible. This can therefore be classed as a lymphocytic leukaemia.
(c) In spite of the severe and acute nature of the condition, the normal lymphocyte morphology is a good prognostic sign for response to chemotherapy in the short to medium term. Cases of prolymphocytic and lymphoblastic leukaemia are generally unresponsive to chemotherapy: however, the prospects for attainment of remission in lymphocytic leukaemia are reasonably good. Unfortunately, long-term prognosis is still bad, as remission seldom lasts for more than about 18 months, and is sometimes considerably shorter. It is therefore necessary to discuss the situation sensitively with the owner and to decide whether or not to embark on treatment according to the individual circumstances of the case.

227 (a) Iritis.

(b) A small pupil (miosis), congestion of blood vessels on the surface of the iris, hyphaema, and keratitis precipitata.

(c) Toxoplasmosis, feline infectious peritonitis, multicentric lymphosarcoma, and FIV.

228 (a) Iatrogenic infective arthritis. The usual organisms are staphylococci, strepto-cocci, coliforms, *Pseudomonas* and clostridia.

(b) Initially, an increased soft tissue density representing a joint effusion. Later, the joint space becomes narrowed as the articular cartilage is destroyed. When the infection enters the subchondral bone, a mixture of bone lysis and new bone formation is seen.

(c) Culture the organism and identify its antibiotic sensitivity. Samples may be obtained by synoviocentesis or biopsy of the synovial membrane. Vigorous joint lavage, with or without synovectomy, combined with the administration of a suitable systemic anti-biotic, should be the first line of treatment. If extensive damage has occurred, and the joint remains persistently painful after the infection has been controlled, it may be necessary to perform an arthrodesis.

229 (a) Lactation in the non-pregnant and pregnant bitch is associated with the fall in plasma progesterone concentration which occurs at about 50 days after ovulation. This fall in progesterone stimulates the release of prolactin which initiates lactation. In the present case, ovariectomy has removed the source of progesterone production and resulted in a rapid decline of plasma concentrations. This could have been avoided by performing surgery when progesterone concentrations are normally low (after the end of metoestrus, i.e. more than 70 days after the end of oestrus).

(b) Conservative therapy may be successful, but many cases require further treatment. Hormonal preparations (progestagens, androgens, oestrogens, and a combination of the latter two) may all be used to suppress pituitary release of prolactin. The progestagens commonly employed include megestrol acetate and proligestone. These are usually successful, although sometimes it is necessary to 'wean' bitches off therapy slowly since abrupt termination of drug administration may potentiate a further release of prolactin. In recurrent cases a specific prolactin antagonist such as bromocriptine may be administered. If ovarian tissue has been left in the bitch after ovariohysterectomy, signs of oestrus will be seen.

230 (a) Assessment of pain in animals is difficult, but behavioural patterns (the cat being reluctant to move and remaining hunched up at the back of the cage) give an indication. In the absence of evidence that the cat is **not** in pain, it is better to give analgesia following any invasive surgery.

(b) Opioids may be safely and effectively used in cats so long as the doses are not excessive and the drugs are not given by the intravenous route (when excitement may occur). Examples of suitable analgesics are pethidine (meperidine) (1–2 mg/kg intramuscularly) and buprenorphine (0.006 mg/kg intramuscularly), but many other opioid drugs have been satisfactorily used. Non-steroidal anti-inflamatory analgesics (NSAIDs) do not give effective analgesia in severe post-operative pain, but can be very effective where pain results from swelling. NSAIDs are eliminated slowly and are liable to be toxic in cats, but doses of phenylbutazone of 10 mg/kg per day, or aspirin, 25 mg/kg alternate days, have been used safely in this species.

231 (a) Third-degree atrioventricular block.
(b) Try a parasympatholytic drug, e.g. atropine or glycopyrolate; if no response, as is likely, the only worthwhile option is a pacemaker, but the prognosis depends on what underlying heart condition has caused the arrhythmia and whether there is intercurrent disease of other systems.

232 (a) The most likely cause is a fibrocartilaginous embolus causing ischaemia of the spinal cord. A Hansen type I prolapsed intervertebral disc is less likely given the type of dog and the peracute onset of signs.
(b) Intravenous dexamethasone (2 mg/kg body weight twice daily for 48 hours) should be administered. Ancilliary therapy should consist of cage rest and good nursing.
(c) The prognosis is guarded with approximately 50% of cases failing to recover. Those cases that do improve generally show signs of recovery within 10 days. Dogs showing lower motor signs have a poorer prognosis than those showing upper motor signs. Those with a unilateral lesion have a better prognosis.

233 (a) Dental caries (decay) in dogs usually occurs in areas where food and bacterial deposits stagnate, in the occlusal pits and fissures of the posterior teeth. A diet rich in refined carbohydrates, like chocolates and sugar, can encourage decay.
(b) If the cavity is minimal a filling may be placed, but if extensive, extraction of the tooth offers the most sensible treatment.

234 (a) Vitiligo.
(b) Alopecia areata, Vogt-Koyanagi-Harada-like syndrome, and discoid lupus erythematosus.

235 (a) This anaemia is clearly haemolytic. It is regenerative, and not only is there no evidence of haemorrhage, the raised bilirubin is strongly indicative of red cell breakdown. If haemolysis had been less obvious it would perhaps have been necessary to check for signs of hidden haemorrhage (faecal occult blood, paracentesis to check for free blood in the abdomen), as not all cases are easy to differentiate on laboratory results alone. Auto-immune haemolytic anaemia (AIHA) is almost certainly the diagnosis in this case. The bitch is in the peak age group for auto-immune disorders and these are more common in the female. Although there is neutrophilia and pyrexia, these are commonly seen in AIHA as a consequence of red blood cells (RBC) breakdown: this bitch was not really ill enough for an acute infectious haemolysis, and cases of *Leptospira icterohaemorrhagiae* infection are usually markedly jaundiced with high liver enzymes.
(b) A direct Coombs test to demonstrate the presence of antibody-coated red cells is probably the most specific test; an indirect Coombs test to demonstrate the presence of incomplete antibodies in the plasma is also useful in this context. However, 'false' negatives can occur, especially if a dog has been given corticosteroids before testing; if all other indications suggest AIHA, it should not be ruled out simply on the basis of a negative Coombs result.
(c) Treatment of this condition is with high (immunosuppressive) doses of corticosteroids. Prednisolone, given orally at 1 mg/kg *b.i.d.*, is the usual regime; it is important to ensure that this dose level is adhered to, as smaller doses often fail to have the desired effect. Antibiotic cover should also be given. It may be necessary to continue treatment for 10 days or more before the condition goes into remission, and the patient may appear somewhat Cushingoid as a result; however, the dose rate can be gradually

reduced as soon as the PCV has returned to normal, and serious side-effects are unusual. Blood transfusion is frequently stated in text books as being contra-indicated, but in practice problems seem to be quite rare so long as the prednisolone is started before the transfusion. Certainly, it is a risk worth taking if the patient appears likely to die of the anaemia before the prednisolone has had a chance to take effect. If no response has occurred after 10–14 days on prednisolone, azathioprine is recommended as the next thing to try.

(d) Prognosis is good, as the majority of cases attain remission with few problems. Relapse is quite common, but again response to treatment is usually good. Repeated relapses may be treated by maintenance on a low dose of prednisolone or by splenectomy (the spleen is the main site of the haemolysis).

The patient gave a positive result on a direct Coombs test and prednisolone treatment was begun immediately, with ampicillin as a precaution against secondary infection. However, 2 days later the PCV had fallen to 0.08 and the RBC picture was less regenerative. Four hundred and fifty millilitres of blood was collected in ACD from another (unrelated) dog owned by the same family, and this was administered intravenously. Clinical improvement was immediate and the PCV rose to 0.19. The dog's RBC picture, 8 days after the start of treatment, became much more regenerative with many nucleated RBCs in circulation, and 4 days later the PCV had reached 0.38. Prednisolone was gradually reduced over the next 3 weeks and then withdrawn. At a check-up 1 month after finishing treatment the PCV was 0.47, and the bitch remains well.

236 (a) Chemosis or conjunctival oedema.
(b) Microbiological examinations for chlamydia, a known cause in this species.
(c) Eye ointment or drops containing tetracycline ten to twelve times daily.

237 (a) Laryngeal paralysis in dogs shows well-recognised breed, age and sex predispositions. Dogs in the bodyweight range 25–35 kg are most susceptible, and in the United Kingdom the labrador, Afghan hound and Irish setter are the breeds most prone. Dogs are more liable to develop the condition than bitches by a ratio of 2:1. Most affected dogs are over 10 years of age.

Stridorous respiration which may be episodic at first, a moist retching cough and muting of the bark are the most common symptoms reported, but owners may be unaware of a progressive exercise intolerance in an elderly dog. Cyanosis and collapse may occur in advanced cases, and severe hyperthermia can develop in hot weather.

The additional diagnostic procedures which are helpful include:
  (i) General neurological examination.
  (ii) Palpation of the throat.
  (iii) Chest radiography.
  (iv) Laryngoscopy to assess laryngeal function.

Laryngeal paralysis is the dominant feature of a generalised axonopathy. Thus, a full neurological examination is indicated, paying particular attention to hind limb proprioception. In a small number of dogs the decision to perform surgery will be reversed if other neurological deficits are present.

Palpation of the throat serves to eliminate the presence of masses which could be compressing the airway or infiltrating the recurrent nerves. Light pressure on the dorsal aspect of the larynx in cases of paralysis reliably increases the volume of stridor.

Chest radiographs are necessary to eliminate the possibility that an anterior mediastinal mass is causing dysfunction of the recurrent nerves.

Direct laryngoscopy under light anaesthesia confirms the diagnosis (*Figure 267*). The absence of active abductory **and** adductory movements indicates paralysis. Other laryngeal conditions such as chondritis or neoplasia may be seen at this time (*Figure 268*).

(b) The preferred surgical treatments for laryngeal paralysis are collectively known as 'tie-back' operations. Their aim is to fix one of the arytenoid cartilages in an abducted position (*Figure 269*) and they are both effective and relatively free of complications. Note that, although clinical laryngeal paralysis of dogs is a bilateral condition, a unilateral remedy is adequate for the respiratory demands of elderly dogs.

238 Anaesthetic gases in the operating theatre may be reduced by decreased production, or by removing waste gases. Where suitable, both methods should be employed. By far the most effective method of preventing pollution of the operating theatre is that of active scavenging, where expired gases are actively drawn out of the room. Volatile gases may be adsorbed by activated charcoal, but the canisters must be changed regularly, and this method does not remove nitrous oxide. The use of closed circuits, particularly with in-circle vaporisers, reduces the amount of anaesthetic vapour produced. Vaporisers should be filled outside the working area, as it is difficult to avoid spillage.

239 (a) The bitch almost certainly has haemorrhagic gastroenteritis, an acute condition of unknown aetiology. Diagnosis is based on the clinical signs and the absence of other existing causes. There is a striking rise in packed cell volume ($<60\%$) due to fluid loss into the gastrointestinal tract. The age, vaccination status of the animal, and the absence of pyrexia, make parvovirus infection unlikely; canine coronavirus infection is rarely this severe.

(b) Treatment is based on rapid replacement of fluids using balanced electrolyte solutions, with corticosteroids being given if initial response to therapy is poor. Recovery is usually seen in 24–48 hours; failure to do so should prompt investigation of other possibilities, such as foreign bodies.

240 (a) The petechial haemorrhages on the head and elbow joints are indicative of 'red leg', a bacterial infection caused by *Aeromonas hydrophila*, and is the correct diagnosis in this case.

(b) The condition can be treated by administration, orally or by injection, of an appropriate antibiotic. Affected amphibians should be isolated and close attention paid to hygiene.

241 (a) The root of the lower canine was perforated in the plating of a mandibular fracture. The operator was unaware of the dental anatomy and the position of the roots. Chronic osteomyelitis has resulted.

(b) Extraction of the tooth is necessary.

242 (a) Urethral prolapse.

(b) The owner's main complaint concerned the bleeding from the prepuce; however, he might also have noticed the dog licking the area excessively.

(c) The condition is best treated by amputation of the prolapse and suturing urethral urothelium to penile integument circumferentially at the exterrnal urethral orifice, using fine synthetic absorbable material.

243 Many breeders consider that bacteria (especially beta haemolytic streptococci) present within the vagina may result in infertility. However, there is no evidence that vaginal bacterial swab results indicate bacterial colonisation of the uterus. Also, detailed investigations demonstrate aerobic bacteria within the vagina of normal fertile bitches as well as those which are infertile or have a vaginal discharge. The possible significance of anaerobic bacteria has not been elucidated. Bacteriological examination of a bitch with a clinical discharge may reveal overgrowth of one pathogenic bacterium, but the routine pre-breeding swabbing of bitches is of little value. The preputial cavity of male dogs, likewise, has a normal bacterial flora.

244 (a) Second-degree atrioventricular block with a variable PR interval from 0.12–0.2 seconds (Mobitz type I or Wenckebach's phenomenon).

(b) Stop the digoxin tablets to see if the rhythm returns to normal and advise weight reduction (provided no other clinical abnormalities are found).

245 The majority of bitches have their first oestrus between 7 and 14 months of age. However, some normal bitches may not cycle until they reach 2½ years. Failure to cycle at the anticipated time causes considerable concern to the owner. In this example, following the elimination of systemic and nutritional diseases, it should be recommended that the bitch is left for a further 6 months. Contact with oestrous bitches is considered useful by some workers. If there is no response, attempts may be made to induce oestrus. This is time-consuming, expensive, and rarely results in live pups. The induced oestrus is unlike a spontaneous oestrus, and vaginal cytology and plasma progesterone determinations are required to determine the optimal mating time. Oestrus may be induced by the subcutaneous administration of 20 iu/kg equine chorionic gonadotrophin daily for 5 days, with 500 iu (total dose) of human chorionic gonadotrophin given intramuscularly on the fifth day. The latter injection is extremely painful. Luteal function may be inadequate after oestrus-induction.

246 (a) Labial stomatitis in dogs is often mistaken for periodontal disease, although in older animals there may be an overlap in the clinical picture. Some breeds are more prone and there are strong indications that genetic factors play an important role in this condition. The ulcerations invariably occur at the pressure points lying over the upper canines and the premolar teeth.

(b) Antibiotics and oral hygiene regime often prove disappointing as long-term therapy. Extraction of the teeth associated with the ulcerations in severe cases will usually improve the condition, however.

247   The flexed lateral view of the right elbow seen in *Figure 194's* X-ray demonstrates a substantial free triangular bone fragment caudal to the joint, and separated from the ulna by an irregular cleavage line. The fragment is remodelling but as yet there is minimal evidence of secondary degenerative joint disease.

Diagnosis: ununited anconeus; a manifestation of osteochondrosis commonly seen in German shepherd dogs. The opposite elbow should also be X-rayed as the condition is frequently bilateral.

248   (a) The peroneal or fibular nerve.
(b) Loss of skin sensation to the dorsal aspect of the lower leg, hock and paw.
(c) Electromyography of the muscles innervated by the peroneal nerve, e.g. the cranial tibialis and the digital extensor muscles will demonstrate spontaneous electrical activity. Nerve conduction velocity studies would indicate reduced or absent conduction.

249   (a) The red cell picture is moderately regenerative with some polychromatophilic nacrocytes and hypochromasia, particularly in the polychromatophilic cells (the crenation is a result of the smear having been made from a postal sample). Many platelets are visible in this field.
(b) The regenerative nature of the red cell picture effectively rules out hypoplastic/ aplastic anaemia, leaving the alternatives of haemorrhage or haemolysis. The findings which mark this as a chronic haemorrhagic anaemia are the hypochromasia and hypoalbuminaemia (indicative of loss of blood constituents from the body, and only chronic blood loss will produce hypochromasia), and the thrombocytosis is also a feature of the presence of a bleeding point. If blood is being lost from the body and yet there is no obvious clinical evidence of haemorrhage, the intestinal tract is the most likely site. The slightly raised urea is consistent with this, as the subsequent digestion of blood lost into the intestine appears to have the same effect as a high-protein meal in raising plasma urea. The neutrophilia and monocytosis suggest an infected lesion. Thus all the findings point to an infected, chronically bleeding lesion in the (small?) intestine. In a 9-year-old Boxer such a lesion is probably neoplastic.
(c) If the above hypothesis is correct, melaena is probably present and a faecal occult blood test will be positive. This is therefore the first test to perform. Abdominal radiography, especially a barium series, may help visualise the lesion further, but if the faecal occult blood is positive an exploratory laparotomy will be necessary. The whole length of the intestine must be inspected carefully as some lesions are not readily obvious from the serosal surface.
In this case, a faecal occult blood test was positive and an exploratory laparotomy was performed the following day. After careful inspection a small vascular tumour (about 1 cm diameter) was identified in the jejunum. A 10 cm section of jejunum including the tumour was resected, and the lesion was later identified histologically as a leiomyosarcoma. Post-operative recovery was uneventful. A marked clinical improvement was reported by the owner 10 days after surgery, and the PCV had increased to 0.41. The dog remains well.

250   (a) Bacterial cheilitis.
(b) *Staphylococcus aureus*.
(c) This lesion is commonly associated with poor-quality abrasive foodstuffs.

251 There are pale feathers as well as the normal black ones. Colour changes in feathers can be due to: (i) Normal maturation of plumage as the bird becomes adult. (ii) A nutritional deficiency. (iii) A viral infection affecting feather growth and development. This bird had psittacine beak and feather disease (PBFD).

252 (a) Salivary cysts may arise in one or more of three sites in the dog. In order of frequency, these are:
   (i) Cervical (*Figure 270*).
   (ii) Sublingual (ranula or 'honey cyst') (*Figure 271*).
   (iii) Intermediate (pharyngeal) (*Figure 272*).
(b) The cause of salivary cysts is not known other than that a leakage develops from one of the small ducts leading between the lobules of the monostomatic section of the sublingual gland and the main sublingual duct itself. The parotid, mandibular and infra-orbital glands are virtually never involved in salivary cysts. Leaked saliva gathers in the fascial planes and, because it is mildly irritant, a layer of inflammatory reactive tissue forms giving the impression of a cyst wall. However, this layer is not secretory and its removal is ineffective as a treatment for a salivary cyst. In a small number of dogs, bilateral cysts develop simultaneously. Otherwise, the side of origin is not difficult to determine in the early stages. However, cervical salivary cysts tend to migrate by gravity towards the ventral midline as they enlarge, and, hopefully, owners will remember where they began! The side of origin will be obvious when the cyst is sublingual or pharyngeal. In cats, salivary cysts are invariably sublingual (*Figure 273*). The presenting signs of pharyngeal cysts often relate to the dyspnoea or dysphagia which a mass in the paratonsillar region would cause.
(c) Surgical removal of the source of the saliva, i.e. the sublingual chain, is the only effective remedy. Simultaneous excision of the mandibular gland is also necessary, since it shares a common capsule with the sublingual gland.

253 (a) Follicular conjunctivitis.
(b) The presence of small follicles on the palpebral conjunctiva, often causing depigmentation in affected places.

254 (a) The radiograph seen in *Figure 200* is consistent with a diagnosis of **rupture of the diaphragm**. Note the presence of gas-filled viscera in the thorax.
(b) The immediate priorities are:
   (i) **Stabilisation of any hypovolaemic shock** (caused by pulmonary or intrathoracic haemorrhage), while carefully avoiding the over-administration of fluids which may add to any pulmonary oedema.
   (ii) Management of possible hypoxia by **oxygen administration** (e.g. via face mask, oxygen tent, nasal entubation, tracheostomy tube).
   (iii) **Monitoring cardiac function** for signs of arrhythmias resulting from myocardial contusion.
(c) The condition should be resolved by **surgical repair** of the diaphragm at laparotomy. This should be performed once the animal is stable, allowing any pulmonary or myocardial contusions to resolve. The ideal time for this is therefore 5–7 days after the trauma. (Surgery in the first few days after trauma is associated with an increased risk of morbidity due to possible lung or myocardial pathology; and beyond the first week, it may be complicated by the presence of intra-thoracic adhesions.)

255 This cat had a severe pneumothorax and would be very hypoxic. Ideally, **no drugs** should be used before the chest is drained, as respiratory depression, or even lateral recumbency, may cause death. However, if the cat becomes further distressed, increased oxygen consumption can also cause death.

(a) Radiography adequate for diagnosis is often possible by restraining the cat in a box (as was done in this case).

(b) Ideally, the chest should be drained using local anaesthesia, but while this can be done in dogs, cats may become distressed. If chemical restraint is required, a method of 'minimal interference' to 'maximal support' should be employed. With the surgeon ready to drain the chest, anaesthesia is induced with a rapidly acting intravenous agent, and the cat ventilated with 100% oxygen (by mask) until some air has been withdrawn from the pleural cavity, at which stage the immediate emergency is over, and the cat can be intubated.

256 (a) Purulent feline stomatitis.

(b) The cause is most likely to be a systemic immuno-depressed reaction. Some connection with viral infection has been demonstrated but not positively proven in all cases.

(c) Systemic corticosteroids and antibiotics, as well as early extraction of all the involved teeth, may improve the condition, but the prognosis is usually poor.

257 The size, shape and position of the prostate gland may be determined using plain radiography and contrast studies. Involvement of local lymph nodes may also be demonstrated. Real-time B-mode ultrasound provides additional information about the prostatic architecture; this may be particularly useful in cases of paraprostatic cysts. Perirectal or transabdominal needle biopsy of the prostate allows its histological examination. However, if abscessation is suspected, tissue collection should be attempted at laparotomy.

Bacterial isolation from the third (prostatic) fraction of the ejaculate, and collection of prostatic fluid by aspiration from the urethra during prostatic massage, may provide useful information – although bacteria may be found in some normal dogs, too.

258 (a) Litters of kittens with persistent conjunctivitis in the absence of other overt signs of upper respiratory tract disease are likely to be infected with feline *Chlamydia psittaci*. Feline calicivirus (FCV) and feline herpes virus, though they may affect young kittens in vaccinated colonies, invariably cause nasal discharge, sneezing and, in the case of FCV, oral ulceration in addition to conjunctivitis. The queen is almost certainly a symptomless carrier and source of infection. Diagnosis of *C. psittaci* can be made by demonstration of the organism on conjunctival scrapings or on culture, but both require specialised facilities.

(b) Response to treatment with systemic tetracyclines given over a 3-week period is usually diagnostic, though in kittens the use of tetracycline may be contra-indicated as the drug causes discolouration of teeth. Chloramphenicol, though effective, is usually avoided due to its haemopoietic effects, and in such circumstances erythromycin may be the drug of choice. Local application of antibiotics via eye drops is ineffective in maintaining therapeutic levels unless carried out multiple (*c.* 12) times a day.

259 (a) The main abnormalities are a slight to moderate non-regenerative anaemia and a very marked neutropenia. This does tend to suggest a degree of bone marrow suppression, but on the other hand not all bone marrow cell lines are affected. The neutropenia, in particular, is very suggestive of some sort of viral infection.

(b) The two main differential diagnoses are FeLV and FIV, with the emphasis on the latter because of the cat's lifestyle, which puts him in a high-risk FIV category, and the neutropenia, which is often a feature of this condition.

(c) Serological testing for evidence of one or both of these viruses would be the next step.

(d) It is always upsetting to have to recommend euthanasia when an animal is not apparently seriously ill, and in cases like this it is not always necessary. So long as reasonable precautions can be taken to minimise the chances of the infection being passed on to other cats, FIV-positive animals may continue with a reasonable quality of life for quite some time after diagnosis. As this cat's lifestyle was the means of acquiring FIV infection, it is likely to be the means of passing it on. If he can be prevented from roaming, fighting and copulating he will become much less of a danger to feline society, and any illnesses he develops can be treated as they occur. With this aim in mind neutering would be extremely advisable, after which attempts to keep him at home might have some hope of success.

This cat was initially given a 10-day course of amoxycillin, after which the abscess had completely resolved, rectal temperature was normal, and the respiratory sounds were less harsh. The owner had previously rejected all advice regarding neutering for apparently anthropomorphic reasons, but gave his permission when the situation regarding transmission of FIV was explained. Fortunately, there were no other cats in the household. The cat was admitted for castration and teeth scaling.

260 (a) Eosinophilic granuloma (EG).

(b) The aetiology of this complex of diseases is not understood and it is therefore not surprising that a number of empirical treatments are advocated. However, if the cause is not known logical therapy cannot be applied and none of the recommended remedies has a high level of success. Immunomodulation with corticosteroids, oral megoestrol acetate, surgical excision, cryosurgery and radiotherapy all have their supporters.

The labial form of EG is sometimes known as 'rodent ulcer', but this is a term best avoided because a condition with the same label occurs in man, where it is used to describe facial basal cell carcinoma. Labial EG is sometimes accompanied by lesions on the palate and dorsal surface of the tongue. Other sites which can be involved in this syndrome include the trunk (plaque form) and the limbs (linear form).

261 (a) Trichomoniasis ('frounce') is the most common cause of stomatitis in birds of prey.

(b) The protozoon parasite is often acquired from pigeons.

262 Vaginal cytology can be examined using the facilities of a practice laboratory. Samples of vaginal fluid can be collected by aspiration using a shortened bovine inseminating pipette. Smears should then be made (see *Figures 274–277*); these can be stained by a Leishman's or any other stain used for blood smears. Examination of the smears for the maximum degree of epithelial cell cornification will allow identification of the best mating time. At this stage there are usually no neutrophils present and the background of the smear is relatively clear of debris, although bacteria may be numerous, as are ethyrocytes. It is also useful to monitor the peripheral plasma concentrations of progesterone; these increase in the bitch a few days prior to ovulation. Measurements can be made on alternate days using an enzyme-linked immunoassay (ELISA) test kit.

263 (a) A biologically active (hypertrophic) non-union of the olecranon.

(b) The distractive force generated by the triceps muscle was not counteracted by a tension band. The minor rotational and bending forces should be controlled with two Kirschner wires, while the major distractive force should be converted into a compressive force at the fracture site by the application of a figure-of-eight wire placed on the caudal aspect of the ulna.

(c) Since the non-union is biologically active it should heal if it is compressed – see (b). Curettage of the fracture site is not indicated but it may be packed with autogenous cancellous bone to encourage healing.

264 (a) The ECG (*Figure 206*) shows ventricular pre-excitation. PR intervals are short, with a 'delta' wave in leads II, III and aVF. The mean elecrical axis in the frontal plane is $+10°$, i.e. there is left axis deviation, and the QRS complexes are very wide (0.1 sec). The rate and rhythm are normal at the time of the recording.

(b) Pre-excitation is a situation where supraventricular impulses bypass all or part of the atrioventricular nodes via accessory pathways, and this may result in paroxysmal tachycardia because of re-entry through retrograde conduction. During these periods of very rapid heart rate, the dog may appear distressed or actually collapse. In this dog the condition is probably congenital.

(c) The Wolff-Parkinson-White syndrome.

(d) Lignocaine may be effective but is not suitable for daily use. Quinidine, procainamide, tocainide, propranolol and calcium channel blockers have all been suggested. Amiodarone is often used in humans. Digoxin is not recommended because it may accelerate conduction in the accessory pathway.

265 (a) Epiphora.

(b) Imperforate punctum, particularly in this breed. Other causes include blockage of the nasolacrimal duct system by mucus or purulent material or possibly a foreign body.

(c) Examination with magnification to find if a punctum is present and/or irrigation of the nasolacrimal duct system via a cannula in the upper punctum.

266 (a) This is egg peritonitis with the presence of yolk material around the oviducts and non-shelled ova.

(b) The shelled eggs are in the urinary bladder, which is a very thin-walled structure (the Allis tissue forceps are tearing it). The eggs are able to pass into the bladder in debilitated or dystokic chelonia because the bladder and oviducts open into a common cloaca. Eggs in the cloaca which are not expelled will occasionally move cranially into the bladder. This is facilitated in chelonia by the virtual absence of a urethra, the bladder opening directly into the cloaca.

267 *Figure 209* shows a kinked endotracheal tube, and *Figure 210* a tube obstructed by over-inflation of the cuff. In *209*, the obstruction is almost total, and the dog either would have stopped breathing, or would be making major respiratory efforts which did not result in movement of the reservoir bag. Obstruction could have been prevented by using an 'armoured' tube which has a spiral support in the wall. In *Figure 210* the obstruction is incomplete, but would lead to a fall in arterial oxygen (significant if the cat was breathing air, but less so if it was receiving oxygen supplementation) and to a rise in arterial carbon dioxide (hypercarbia). Hypercarbia causes tachynoea, muscle twitches (often incorrectly interpreted as lightening of anaesthesia), and bright red mucous membranes, and the heart may be sensitised to arrhythmic effects of circulating adrenaline. Care must be taken not to over-pressurise the cuff; in this case (a cat), the problem could have been avoided by using an uncuffed tube.

Figure 211 shows an endotracheal tube which has been advanced too far, and is probably in one bronchus. Chest movement might be uneven, but the major symptoms result from the failure of the non-aerated lung lobes to excrete carbon dioxide or to take up the volatile anaesthetics. Signs of hypercarbia would be seen, and the levels of volatile agent required for anaesthesia would be higher than expected. The problem can be avoided by cutting the endotracheal tubes to a suitable length before the animal is anaesthetised.

Figure 212 shows a broken endotracheal tube loose in the airway. If this had been left, symptoms would have ranged from a chronic cough to the death of the animal. It could have been avoided by the earlier removal of the endotracheal tube. The time of removal of the tube is controversial, however. Early removal leaves the animal's airway unprotected, but leaving the tube in place until laryngeal reflexes return risks situations such as that illustrated in *Figure 212*, and, more commonly, may cause laryngeal damage to the cat, and discomfort to the dog. Where endotracheal tubes are required until laryngeal reflexes return (e.g. brachiocephalic dogs which obstruct when conscious), a secure gag should be used to prevent the tube (or the nurse) from being bitten.

268 This dog is losing blood from the urethra between micturitions. However, the blood could have originated from the penis or prepuce, and so these areas should be examined first. Urethral haemorrhage in male dogs may originate in the urethra (e.g. secondary to trauma or neoplasia), but the associated lesions usually also result in dysuria. If preputial/penile bleeding is absent, a more likely site of origin for the haemorrhage is the prostate gland. This particular dog is suffering from idiopathic prostatic haemorrhage.

269 (a) All of them. A thorough examination of the skin as a whole is a major component of the initial assessment of all dogs with otitis externa. This is likely to be especially rewarding when the otitis is bilateral. Canine otology should be regarded as a branch of dermatology and the need to perform surgery on the ear is an admission of failure to control dermatoses.

(b) *Figure 214* shows contact allergic dermatitis. Other areas with poor hair cover, i.e. the ventral aspect of the abdomen and the interdigital webs, showed inflammatory changes. *Figure 215* shows verrucose otitis due to chronic atopy. Both areas were similarly afflicted. The ears were highly pruritic from the outset. Self-induced lesions were present elsewhere on the body.

270 The heart base and trachea are depressed by an elongated gas-filled structure running through the dorsal thorax. Caudal to the heart, the dorsal and ventral walls of this structure are visible as thin radiodense lines. The lung fields show a patchy increase in density (alveolar pattern), especially in the cranial lobes, and there are increased bronchial markings. Minor thoracic spondylosis is an incidental finding.

Diagnosis: acquired megaoesophagus with secondary inhalation pneumonia. The dilated oesophagus is clearly visible and a barium study is not indicated.

271 (a) Ununited, or fragmented, coronoid process.

(b) A medial elbow arthrotomy, either retracting or transecting the pronator teres and flexor carpi radialis muscles. The medial collateral ligament of the elbow may be sectioned to improve accesss.

(c) The other forms of osteochondrosis seen in the elbow are osteochondritis dissecans of the medial humeral condyle, ununited anconeal process and ununited medial epicondyle.

272 Bitches with pyometritis are toxaemic, and are often fluid-deficient from losses via the kidney, and from vomiting. Fluid therapy should be instituted and at least the circulating volume restored prior to premedication and anaesthesia. Anaesthetic drugs should be chosen so as to have minimal effects on the cardiovascular system, and to ensure a rapid recovery. Careful monitoring is necessary, and this and fluid therapy must be continued throughout anaesthesia and the recovery period.

273 (a) Perineal rupture with retroflexion of the bladder into the perineum (N.B. this is not always associated with dysuria).

(b) The immediate management is non-surgical. The dysuria must be relieved. Catheterisation is not usually possible, so the bladder should be drained by needle centesis via the perineum. The empty bladder can then often be returned by pressure on the perineum to the abdomen and a urethral catheter passed. If so, the catheter should be maintained *in situ* until the metabolic effects of the dysuria have been corrected by appropriate fluid and electrolyte therapy. Surgical repair of the perineal defect can then be performed, but earlier surgical intervention is indicated if the bladder distension cannot be relieved, and the bladder returned to the abdomen and a urethral catheter passed.

274 (a) Fracture of the crown exposing the pulp which is still vital and free of infection.

(b) The most suitable treatment would be a pulpotomy using a calcium hydroxide dressing. At this age the root canal is large and its apical foramen may be too divergent for a well-condensed root filling. As the blood supply to the pulp is still excellent calcium hydroxide can encourage the formation of a reparative dentine bridge. By walling off the exposure and maintaining the vitality of the pulp, the development of the root formation may progress to maturity.

275 (a) Anaesthesia for caesarian section requires anaesthesia of the dam adequate for surgical and humanitarian requirements with minimal effects on the young when they are delivered. Ideally, the dam should have a rapid painfree recovery so that she can nurse the offspring. Many methods of anaesthesia have been successfully used. There are two possible approaches, these being the use of drugs which will be rapidly eliminated, and the use of drugs which have antagonists and can be reversed.

The use of volatile agents to induce and maintain anaesthesia results in the least residual drug in the young. However, prior to maintenance with volatile agents minimal doses of short-acting intravenous induction agents may be used, propofol being particularly successful provided an adequate time (20 minutes) is allowed for its elimination before delivery. Saffan has been successfully used in the cat; kittens do remain sleepy but respiratory depression is minimal.

Drugs with specific antagonists are opioids and the alpha 2 adrenoceptor agonists. Neither are adequate for surgery on their own, and the other component of combinations used will not be reversed. Opioids are usually combined with sedatives, often as commercially prepared combinations such as etorphine/methotrimeprazine. Relapse into sedation can occur. Medetomidine has been used in combination with very low doses of volatile anaesthetic agents for caesarian section. A point to consider is that antagonists will also antagonise the analgesic effects of the original drugs.

(b) During anaesthesia for caesarian section vomiting may be a real danger. When the dam is recumbent, pressure of the full uterus on the lungs causes hypercarbia and reduced uptake of volatile agents, and pressure on the vena cava may prevent venous return, leading to cardiovascular collapse. Post-operative bleeding may also occur.

276 (a) The most likely diagnosis is fibrous osteodystrophy (metabolic bone disease) due to a poor calcium: phosphorus ratio in the diet.
(b) The diagnosis can be confirmed by radiography, which will usually reveal poorly mineralised bones, sometimes associated with pronounced bowing and folding fractures.

277 (a) There is marked right axis deviation and tall P waves (P pulmonale), which suggest right ventricular and right atrial enlargement.
(b) The likely diagnosis would be pulmonic stenosis, causing right ventricular hypertrophy and secondary right atrial enlargement because of tricuspid incompetence.
(c) This can be confirmed by radiography and ultrasound.

278 (a), (c), (f) and (g) are all important. Protein levels in the diet should be restricted and protein of high biological value (i.e. availability) used. Phosphorus levels should be restricted to combat the renal hyperparathyroidism. Additional salt is not necessary and indeed may be harmful, producing hypertension which may in turn exacerbate renal damage. Management of intercurrent disease is important to prevent the addition of a pre-renal component to the underlying renal failure.

279 As a result of the initial obstruction, the increase in intravesical pressure led to bladder wall ischaemia. This is reversible if relieved quickly enough but the duration of the initial episode of dysuria in this cat was sufficient to lead to necrosis of the bladder lining. Part of the lining subsequently sloughed (shown on the swab next to the bladder) and obstructed the bladder neck, causing further dysuria. The sloughed tissue is displaced by a urethral catheter and so may not be detected on catheterisation.

280 (a) Eosinophilic plaques.

(b) Eosinophilic plaques are frequently associated with self-trauma in allergic cats, and the recurrent fur balls are suggestive of excessive grooming, often the only sign of pruritus in the cat.

(c) Removal of any underlying factors and systemic glucocorticoid therapy. Occasionally, surgical intervention is indicated.

281 (a) Enchondrohystrophy of the English Pointer.

(b) Homozygous recessive.

(c) Enchondrodystrophic puppies have widened growth plates similar to those seen in rickets, but their bone density is normal. They may also develop articular changes as they become older.

282 (a) Entropion.

(b) In-turning of the lower lid with consequent irritation due to facial hair rubbing on the cornea, profuse lacrimation, mild corneal opacity in this case and retraction of the globe.

(c) Surgical correction by removal of an elliptical piece of skin.

283 (a) Overall, these results are highly suspicious of FIP. The most important findings in this respect are the hyperglobulinaemia and hypoalbuminaemia. Although slightly/moderately raised globulins are a common non-specific finding in sick cats, high globulins (>70 g/l) combined with low albumin are very characteristic of FIP. The slightly raised liver enzymes and slight icterus are also typical (although **high** liver enzymes and marked jaundice are suggestive more of lymphocytic cholangitis in otherwise similiar circumstances). In spite of the viral nature of the condition, most cases show a mild-to-moderate neutrophilia, and a degree of anaemia is also a common finding.

(b) The most important test at this stage is FIP serology. Other tests such as protein electrophoresis may give interesting peripheral information, but add little to the diagnostic certainty.

(c) Conclusive diagnosis of FIP can be tricky, due to the absence of any specific test to demonstrate the clinical disease. Even strong positive antibody levels can be demonstrated in clinically healthy cats with an immunity to the virus. A reasonable rule of thumb is to assess three criteria as follows:

(i) Typical clinical signs of 'wet' FIP (large amounts of proteinaceous abdominal fluid).

(ii) Classic FIP picture on routine biochemistry and haematology (principally hyperglobulinaemia/hypoalbuminaemia, but usually accompanied by the other findings listed above).

(iii) High FIP antibody levels in either serum or ascitic fluid.

If a cat shows a positive diagnosis of FIP under any two of these three headings, then it is a reasonable conclusion that it is suffering from clinical FIP. Although this cat's clinical signs were not those of classic 'wet' FIP they were reasonably consistent with 'dry' FIP, and the positive findings under both (ii) and (iii) lead to a reasonably certain diagnosis.

284 (a) The age and breed of the dog, and the history and appearance of the faeces, are all typical of maldigestion/malabsorption associated with pancreatic atrophy and insufficiency (EPI). Bacterial overgrowth in the proximal small bowel may cause similar signs, as, less commonly may, eosinophilic or plasma cell/lymphocytic enteritis; however, these generally result in a less severe weight loss and do not lead to the khaki-coloured fatty cowpat-like faeces typical of EPI.

(b) Confirmation of EPI is best made on serum levels of TLI (trypsinogen-like immunoreactivity); faecal trypsin levels are an unreliable indication of pancreatic function, and PABA digestion and absorption following oral administration is a less convenient test. Serum B_{12} and folate levels may be abnormal, associated with secondary bacterial overgrowth, with folate elevated and B_{12} reduced. Such secondary overgrowth probably accounts for the occasional episodes of more profound diarrhoea sometimes seen in cases of EPI.

285 (a) Traumatic pulp exposure has resulted in the natural sequel of pulp death.

(b) Yes. The discoloured hole at the centre of the tooth indicates that the root canal contains necrotic material. This can lead to periapical pathology, pain, localised and regional infections, as well as systemic consequences. Endodontic treatment is the least traumatic solution.

286 (a) This is a case of para-aural abscess (PAA). In *Figure 228* the most obvious sinus tract opens below the lateral canthus of the eye, but another opens in the temporal area. Note that the dog has previously been subjected to a lateral-wall ear resection, and that the additus to the horizontal canal has closed. When surgical seekers are introduced into the sinus tracts, they lead towards the ear (*Figure 278*).

PAA arise when suppuration extends from a blind ear canal into the surrounding soft tissues. This occurs if the canal is obstructed by congenital atresia, inflammatory reactions, or neoplasia. Initially, the abscess will produce a swelling of the parotid area and may be confused with a diseased parotid salivary gland. The sinus tracts which appear later can open at a considerable distance from the ear, as in the example illustrated. Whenever sinus tracts develop on the side of the head, otoscopy should be performed, if only to establish whether or not the ear canal is obstructed.

(b) Treatment of PAA invariably requires removal of the residual ear canal, which should always be performed in conjunction with lateral bulla osteotomy.

287 (a) Candidiasis (*Candida albicans* infection). The 'Turkish towel' appearance of the crop is almost pathognomonic.

(b) Confirmation is by culture and/or histopathological examination.

288 (a) The cat has nephrotic syndrome associated with membranous glomerulonephritis. The diagnosis can be supported by the finding of large quantities of albumin in the urine and hypoalbuminaemia. Hypercholesteraemia is usually present.

(b) Confirmation of the membranous glomerulonephritis requires renal biopsy and demonstration of changes by electron microscopy. Immunofluorescent techniques may be used to confirm the presence of immune complexes, usually containing IgG. Treatment is supportive and the short-term prognosis is good; recurrence may well happen, however, and some cases progress to renal failure.

289 (a) Exophthalmos or proptosis.

(b) Retrobulbar mass, usually either tumour or infection.

(c) Prominence of both globe and nictitating membrane on the affected side, in comparison with the other side, and evidence of lacrimation. Resistance to retropulsion of the globe is another useful diagnostic clinical sign.

290 The most likely potential pathogens to be detected are the protozoon, *Trichomonas gallinae* (the cause of 'pigeon canker'), the yeast, *Candida albicans* and the nematode, *Capillaria contorta*.

291 (a) This is an avulsion fracture of the cranial (anterior) cruciate ligament.

(b) Stifle pain and joint swelling; a positive cranial drawer movement.

(c) The medial meniscus may be damaged in up to 50% of cases, especially where the rupture is chronic.

292 (a) This is a typical case of 'mouthrot' (necrotic stomatitis).

(b) Diagnosis is confirmed by bacteriological examination – gram-negative organisms are usually the cause or involved as secondaries.

(c) Treatment is based on a combination of topical therapy – regular débridement and irrigation with an antiseptic/antibiotic – and systemic antimicrobial agents.

293 (a) The patient is in atrial fibrillation, with a rapid ventricular response rate. This reduces the time available for ventricular filling, which further decreases the cardiac output – which may already be decreased by poor left ventricular function.

(b) The lateral radiograph shows a tall heart with marked left atrial enlargement, and straightening of the caudal border – which suggests left ventricular enlargement, also. The trachea is pushed dorsally and there is increased pulmonary density, particularly in the hilar area, which has the fluffy appearance characteristic of pulmonary oedema. The likely diagnosis is idiopathic giant breed cardiomyopathy.

294 The heart shows marked enlargement for a deep-chested breed. The trachea is elevated, and a large left atrium is visible as a bulge on the caudodorsal margin of the heart. The lung fields show a diffuse mottled increase in density, with some air bronchograms.

Diagnosis: dilated cardiomyopathy with acute pulmonary oedema due to left-sided heart failure.

INDEX

Numbers refer to question and answer numbers.

s